YOGA *for* HEALTH & PERSONALITY

Dr. G. Francis Xavier

PUSTAK MAHAL®

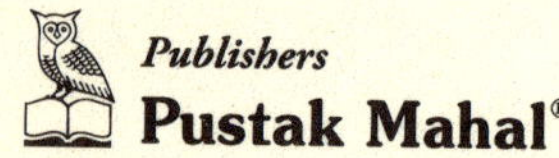

Publishers
Pustak Mahal®

Administrative office and sale centre

J-3/16 , Daryaganj, New Delhi-110002
☎ 23276539, 23272783, 23272784 • *Fax:* 011-23260518
E-mail: info@pustakmahal.com • *Website:* www.pustakmahal.com

Branches
Bengaluru: ☎ 080-22234025 • *Telefax:* 080-22240209
E-mail: pustakmahalblr@gmail.com
Mumbai: ☎ 022-22010941, 022-22053387
E-mail: unicornbooksmumbai@gmail.com
Patna: ☎ 0612-3294193 • *Telefax:* 0612-2302719
E-mail: rapidexptn@gmail.com

© Pustak Mahal, New Delhi

ISBN 978-81-223-0892-1

Edition: 2016

Price : ₹ 195/-

The Copyright of this book, as well as all matter contained herein (including illustrations) rests with the Publishers. No person shall copy the name of the book, its title design, matter and illustrations in any form and in any language, totally or partially or in any distorted form. Anybody doing so shall face legal action and will be responsible for damages.

Printed at : Radha Offset, Delhi

Dedicated to

MY MOTHER

With Love and Respect

Acknowledgement

I owe a debt of gratitude to the following persons from whom I have derived knowledge and experience in Yoga by their personal instructions and/or by reading their books: Swami Gitananda, Swami Poornananda Tirtha, Shri Yogendra, Swami Satyananda Saraswathi, Swami Kuvalayanda, Swami Sivananda, Swami Vivekananda, Rev. Fr. J.M. Dechanet.

I also express my profound gratitude to the following persons for their valuable guidance and support in my literary pursuit, whose names are given below in **alphabetical order**: V. Acharya, Alvin Chua, Prof. Arul Marianathan, T. Amaladas Fernando, Anil B.P., Prof. L. Augustin Amaladas, Ayaz Merali, Babu K. Verghese, Bharath Kapasi, Chandroo, Emmanuel Das, Fred Ochieng, P. Gasper, Gerard Cameons, Mrs. Kalpa Rajesh, G.S.R. Krishna, Mrs. Mala Gerard, Mrs. I. Gunasekar, R. Ilangovan, Ilyas Montri, Isabella Gaha, Most Rev. Dr. Joseph D'Silva, Dr. M. Joseph, Fr. Jayanathan, Msgr. S. Jabamalai, Joseph Victor, K. Jothiramalingam, M. Kandasami, Dr. P. Kansal, V.C. Kumaran, P.N. Kalra, Mrs. Kiran Kuller, M. Kuruvan, M. Mahadeva Raju, M.S. Manjunath, Mrs. Mary Okelo, M.B. Meti, B.E. Naidu, O.P. Narang, P. Narayana Bhat, Sr. Nicola Sprenger, Dr. Pius A. Okelo, Patrick D'Souza, Prakash Gangaram, Rajesh K. Padia, Radhakrishnan, Rajni Shah, P.A. Raj Kumar, S.V. Ramani, Rajiv Beri, K.C. Rangaswamy, E. Ravi Chandran, Dr. J.N. Reddy, Reinhard Sprenger, Roger Khoo, Fr. Ronnie Prabhu, G.P. Shah, Prof. Shanthi Augustin, Shanmuga Verma, Simon Lourdes, R. Sunder Raj, D. Thankaraj, and Vinod Kashyap.

I express my deep indebtedness to Mr. M. Vijaya Kumar, Commissioner of Income Tax, Hyderabad, for writing the Foreword for this book.

I am specially thankful to Mr. Liladhar Bharadia, for the trouble he has taken to arrange the photographs appearing in this book. I also profusely thank Dr. Arvind Pathak and his daughter Poonam Pathak, whose pictures appear in this book along with my postures.

My sincere thanks to Mr. Nigel Fernandes for his continued support in my literary pursuits.

I owe a deep sense of gratitude to my publishers, M/s Pustak Mahal and its Editorial Department for bringing out this book in an excellent manner with meticulous care and diligence.

Last but not the least, my family members for their patience, support and cooperation: my wife Mrs. A. Antoniammal, my children Dr. Denis Xavier, Freeda, Peter, Sheela, and Prakash Xavier, and my grandchildren, Nikita, Alan and Preetika.

Preface

The summer came and with it came the holidays too. I went to my aunt's house and made friends with the young boy there; we went together to the field to feed the cattle.

I was only 11 years of age then. While playing, the young boy surprised me by standing erect on his head. This was the most exciting vacation in my life. I persuaded the boy to teach me the technique of standing 'upside down' without realising that it was the King of Asanas – I was innocently ignorant! But now, as a seasoned Yoga practitioner, I consider the young boy my first 'guru'.

At that time I did not realise that the practice of Yoga improves one's health and personality. Therefore, I did not practise Yoga. Since early childhood onwards, I was a sickly child suffering from a variety of diseases. Only at the age of 37, when I was the Principal of Cooperative Staff Training College, Bangalore, I took to Yoga at the instance of an allopathic physician, Dr Dhananjaya. Within a period of five to six months my health improved considerably.

Thereafter, I took serious interest in Yoga. I spared no pains to learn several tough Yoga techniques from a number of reputed practitioners. Besides the personal instructions and guidance that I received, I equipped myself further by reading as many books and journals as possible.

I have been consistently practising Yoga for many decades and this book is the result of my experiments with Yoga.

Here, I have established a new wave of thought that Yoga has nothing to do with religion. Many Christians and Muslims feel hesitant to take up Yogic practices for fear that Yoga may be against their religious faith. But I have scientifically and logically proved that people of any faith can, without prejudice, practise Yoga to discipline themselves, both in mind and body. There is nothing like Christian Yoga or Hindu Yoga. Yoga is a simple science expounding certain techniques and methods, practised for integrated development of man's entire being – physical, mental and emotional.

It is an acknowledged fact – borne out by my personal experience – that regular and consistent practise of Yoga will provide:

- Scintillating health
- Sharp intellect
- Youthful looks
- Abundant energy
- Emotional maturity
- Calm and serene mind

- Concern for others, and
- Spiritual awareness

What more does a person require in life? So why not start practising Yoga right away? You may ask – How?

Close this book. Keep it aside. Sit erect. Be comfortable and relaxed. Close your eyes. Now, close your mind. Aha! You may wonder: How is this possible? Right! Then, simply sit still for 15 minutes. What should you do during this time? Nothing! Simply do nothing! Open your eyes after the 15th minute only. If you are able to sit calmly and quietly for a period of 15 minutes everyday, you are on the right path to Yogic life.

You may also go ahead with the Yogic practices given in this book. Practise them regularly without a break even for a single day. This may be the only book that offers you, in a single volume, all practical aspects of Yoga – practices of Asanas, Pranayama, Shatkarma and meditation.

Yoga will improve your personality and make you a better human being. Wish you the best of luck in your endeavour to practise Yoga.

—Dr. G. Francis Xavier
Bangalore
Email: gfrancisxavier@yahoo.co.in

Foreword

There is one export of which Indians can be justifiably proud – Yoga. The whole world is amazed with its intricate use in the attainment of a sound mind in a sound body. No doubt, quacks have taken full advantage of the yearning for Yogic knowledge, especially in Western countries. Genuine teachers of Yoga are few and hard to come by. Dr Xavier is one of them. I have the good fortune to be one of his students and have learnt many Yogic techniques to improve my health and personality.

Yoga is purely a scientific system of techniques to develop an integrated personality. For years, Dr Xavier practised this system himself before he began to preach and teach it.

The graded exercises in chapter after chapter – replete with suitable illustrations – will encourage beginners to follow them without difficulty. An impressive Bibliography appended to this book leaves little doubt about Dr Xavier's thoroughness in this field of physical, mental and emotional fitness. He has blended theory and practice in a masterly manner.

It is a matter of pleasure and privilege for me to write a Foreword for this book as I am one of the admirers of Dr Xavier's sterling qualities. He is a man of many parts. I wish him all success in his endeavours to propagate the principles and practices of Yoga all over the world.

I strongly recommend this book with pride and pleasure for the psychosomatic well-being of prospective practitioners.

—M. Vijaya Kumar
Commissioner of Income Tax
Hyderabad

Contents

Part One

The Nature and Scope of Yoga

What is Yoga?

Yoga is the science of **human development**. It is integrated development of man: physical, mental and emotional. It is a **discipline** that enables man to **actualise his potential** to the fullest extent through self-culture and self-education. It expounds certain techniques and methods that would enable man to have union with the Self (the Divine). The constant practise of Yoga gradually helps in developing the virtues of humility and peace of mind, which ultimately enable man to have a peaceful and **cordial relationship with others.**

A lasting development of man requires an alteration of the germ plasm. Such an alteration does not take place by itself in the human organism. **Yoga has evolved several techniques** to create changes in the germ plasm according to the needs and requirements of its practitioners. The ultimate aim of Yoga is the **transformation of a disintegrated personality into a coherent and cohesive being.**

In his book *The Yoga of Concentration*, Swami Gnanananda says: ***"Yoga is a science. It is applied psychology. Not only is it the means to achieve the purpose of life, but it enables one to do anything one wants, even in this world, with great energy and with great benefit to other people."***

This is the reason why both men and women of all age groups should practise Yoga for **all-round development of their personalities.**

Types of Yoga

Swami Vivekananda enunciates four types of Yoga: viz., Karma Yoga, Bhakti Yoga, Jnana Yoga and Raja Yoga.

Karma Yoga is the Yoga of **action** performed unselfishly for the welfare of others. A Karma Yogi is one who works incessantly for the **good of mankind** without any motive. The path of a Karma Yogi is not to get away from the materialistic world but to live within and learn to enjoy the supreme happiness derived from selfless work. Scientists of the modern world could be considered apt examples of **Karma Yogis**. The motivating force behind most **renowned scientists** is **neither money nor fame** but an irresistible desire to discover the truth hidden in the objective world. It is an attitude of the mind that should be developed consciously.

Bhakti Yoga is the Yoga of **love and purity**. It is more suitable for those predisposed to an emotional propensity. When Jesus Christ said "**Love your enemies**", He was preaching Bhakti Yoga. The love of a mother for her child is more a maternal instinct than a gender-based love. But the love between youngsters of both sexes is motivated by the pleasure-seeking instinct. However, true love goes beyond these parameters and pervades entire humanity without any restriction. **Mother Teresa of Calcutta** could be considered a person who practised Bhakti Yoga in its most exalted form. The methods and techniques of Bhakti Yoga are love and affection toward others without any discrimination. It warrants the **elimination of emotions like hatred, jealousy, prejudice, and enmity** from one's mental make-up.

Jnana Yoga is the Yoga of **knowledge and wisdom**. It does not deal with ordinary knowledge of reading, writing and arithmetic, but goes deeper into the knowledge of man, his life after death, the ultimate aim of man's life, the creation of the universe, etc. It is suitable for all those who are endowed with the capacity to **think and analyse** in an **objective manner**. The deeper they contemplate on the nature of man, life after death and creation of the universe, the greater they are convinced that the whole world is *Maya* (illusory) and transitory in nature and wonder at the greatness of God who is the ultimate reality. This type of feeling ultimately makes many renounce the world and lead a life of seclusion. In this way, most **saints and seers** practise Jnana Yoga.

Raja Yoga is the Yoga of **growth and development** through mental discipline. Patanjali is the highest authority on Raja Yoga. Of all the other Yogas, only Raja Yoga has **prescribed eight steps** to practise in a scientific manner for physical, mental and emotional development.

The first step is **Yama** (social virtues) that deals with:

(a) ***Ahimsa*** (non-violence)

(b) ***Sathya*** (truthfulness)

(c) ***Asteya*** (non-stealing)

(d) ***Brahmacharya*** (continence)

(e) ***Aparigraha*** (unselfishness)

The second step is **Niyama** (personal virtues), which insists on:

(f) ***Soucha*** (purity of body and mind)

(g) ***Santosha*** (contentment)

(h) ***Tapas*** (austerity)

(i) ***Swadhyaya*** (self-study and improvement)

(j) ***Ishwara Pranidhana*** (self-surrender to God)

Yama and Niyama could be considered the **Ten Commandments of Yoga** meant for controlling the passions and emotions of a person and thereby paving the way for practise of higher levels of Yoga.

The third step is **Asana, which refers to body postures,** and **physical exercises** to restore and refresh the body by better circulation of blood, more effective breathing and muscular relaxation.

The fourth step is **Pranayama**. It refers to Yogic exercises of **breath control** used to relax the body and thus recharge the body's batteries. Prana is the generalised manifestation of all forces and power in the universe. Pranayama, therefore, refers, to certain exercises through which every part of the body is filled with Prana and from this vital force a certain amount of **power is generated** in the body. Through Pranayama one is able to exert complete control over his body, mind and emotions.

The fifth step is **Prathiyahara**. It is **control of the senses**, the intentional withdrawal from sights, sounds, smells and feelings of the external world, and selective inattention to the senses.

The sixth step is **Dharna**. It is deep, unrestricted, pinpointed **concentration** of the mind on a particular object or idea.

The seventh step is **Dhyana**, which is **meditative awareness**. For instance, there is a steady flow when oil is poured from one vessel to another; when the flow of concentration (Dharna) is uninterrupted, the state that arises is Dhyana (**meditation**).

The last step in Raja Yoga is **Samadhi**, the **highest level** of meditation and the **supreme goal of Yoga**. It is oneness – union with the Self (the Divine). In the state of Samadhi, the body and senses are at rest as if one is asleep but at the same time, the faculties of mind and reason are fully alert, like when one is wide-awake.

Other Types of Yoga

There are some other types of Yoga, which may be considered **minor**.

(a) **Hatha Yoga** – also called Bhahiranga Yoga (**external Yoga**) – aims to conquer bodily life by a complex of postures (Asanas), breath control (Pranayama), cleansing process (Shat Karma) and some other secret practices, such as Bhandas and Mudras. It seeks to heighten the flow of the vital force (Prana) into the body, thereby freeing the body of all impurities and keeping the nervous system unclogged and alert. A Hatha Yogi succeeds in maintaining the strength of his body and youthfulness till a ripe age and develops many supernormal and psychic powers as he progresses in the performance of advanced Hatha Yoga practice. In its pure and simple form, this Yoga deals with external practices of **disciplining the body** to maintain **sound health** and increase longevity.

(b) **Laya Yoga** – also known as **Mantra Yoga**. It is the opposite of Hatha Yoga. The latter concentrates on the body, which is gross, whereas the former deals with the subtle, which is deeper than Hatha. Laya Yoga introduces the techniques of arresting the mind's attention on **internal sound** (Anahata Nada), the mental repetition of a **sound symbol** (generally a select Mantra) in order to tap the potential energy embedded in a human being. Transcendental Meditation developed and propagated worldwide by Maharishi Mahesh Yogi is one of the simplest techniques of Laya Yoga.

(c) **Japa Yoga** deals with chanting a Mantra and is also called Mantra Ycga. It deals with the **science of sound and vibration, which includes chanting, incantations,** and the repetition of sacred formulae that affect the mind, emotions and health. Laya Yoga deals with internal sounds (Anahata Nada), whereas Japa Yoga is based on **chanting Mantras loudly**.

(d) Ajapa Yoga is a **continuation of Japa Yoga**. When Japa Yoga is perfected and the repetition of a Mantra becomes automatic, it is Ajapa Yoga.

(e) Kundalini Yoga: It is said that the **psychic energy** of man lies in the lower abdominal region. This is called Kundalini Shakti and is likened to a serpent coiled at the base of the spine, blocking a fine channel known as the Sushumna, which travels up the spine. When the Kundalini Shakti is awakened, it ascends to join the supreme power at the Sahasrara in the head. The process of awakening Kundalini Shakti through various Yogic practices is called Kundalini Yoga.

Suitable Yoga for Beginners

The aim of all Yoga is to make man disciplined in every respect but they differ only in their approaches and techniques. **Hatha Yoga** is the most **suitable one for beginners**. The practise of Hatha Yoga ensures sound health and tremendous dynamism in a person. This would provide further scope for taking up the advanced practices of Raja Yoga. For the integrated development of one's personality, it is necessary to practise all types of Yoga. The main emphasis should be given to the practise of Asanas, Pranayama, Shat Karma and meditation.

In this book, therefore, an attempt has been made to explain in detail various practices of Hatha Yoga and also to initiate practices of meditation.

Yoga and Spiritual Life

Spiritual life warrants **dedication and detachment**. A person willing to lead such a life should be prepared to sacrifice everything for the sake of humanity at large. It is generally considered that this type of life is possible only when a person is **not married** and leading the life of a sanyasi (**celibate**). There are many Christian priests and nuns and several swamis and sanyasis of different denominations of Hinduism and Buddhism leading a life of celibacy.

When a person remains unmarried, to a great extent he will go against the natural instinct of sex, which is strongly embedded in every individual who is physically potent. Here, Yoga plays a predominant role in bringing about discipline of both body and mind in the lives of those who are leading a life of celibacy. The techniques evolved in Yoga are so advanced that no other system can match them in **sublimating the sexual urge**.

Indian sages and seers evolved Yoga techniques some 6,000 years ago primarily to sublimate the sexual urge, so as to enable them to lead a spiritual life in its most exalted form. The process of sublimation takes place when **sexual energies are transformed into creative power,** which is popularly known in Yogic parlance as the raising of **Kundalini Shakti**.

Sexual energies in the ordinary life pattern convert matter into a living organism through the process of sexual coitus. This might also be expended through masturbation and other sexual avenues. However, sexual energies could be conserved through certain well-defined techniques of Yoga without much tension and anxiety on the part of the individual in restraining sexual urges and thereby enhancing his creative life.

Yoga and Married Life

Yogic practices were originally designed by Indian Yogis to attain spiritual emancipation. Sexual restraint was considered the most important prerequisite for spiritual development. Therefore, it is erroneously held by many that practise of Yoga is meant for sanyasis, saints and seers who are supposed to renounce the world and lead a life of celibacy. It is also believed by many married people that the practise of Yoga ultimately diminishes their sex drive and potential, eventually leading to impotence. This is **not true**.

It has been scientifically proved beyond any iota of doubt that Yoga **does not hamper sexual potential.** Instead, it **revitalises the physical aspect of sex** and also reconditions mental defects arising from one's own feeling of incompetence and an inferiority complex regarding sexual activities. Since Yogic practices **enhance sexual vigour and vitality** there should be no hesitation on the part of married people to practise Yoga.

Yoga and Sex

The mind plays a tremendous role in our life. The urge for sexual activity first and foremost occurs in the mind of a human being. Yoga takes care of the mind. It streamlines the nervous system that is responsible for the physical aspect of sexual life. Hence, practise of Yoga would definitely **contribute in removing any weaknesses in sexual behaviour.**

Removing Sexual Defects

Indolence and lethargy are important causes that shatter physical and mental discipline. To attain efficiency, discipline is a prerequisite. Even to improve sexual efficiency, **discipline is a must**. One who is prone to sloth and lethargy cannot improve sexual potential. Therefore, everyone should endeavour to conquer indolence. Yoga definitely helps in bringing **vitality and dynamism** in a person, which in turn drives away sloth and indolence and thereby improves potential.

Psychosomatic techniques are applied in both Yoga and sex. Both take into consideration the physical, mental and emotional aspects of man. For example, Yoga gives importance to Asanas that are physical in nature. But through the practise of Pranayama and meditation, the mental and emotional nature of man is also substantially enhanced. Similarly, sex undoubtedly deals with the physical aspect in the form of various sex plays culminating in coitus. At the same time, the mental and emotional aspects in the form of love and affection between the married partners should also be given due place in sexual life. Particularly in married life, genuine love and affection between married partners are too important an aspect to be minimised by anybody. If **sincere love** were not exhibited in married life through sexual activities the entire life of married couples would end in despair.

The practise of Yoga will definitely **improve the neuromuscular and psychosomatic machinery.** Yoga generally promotes certain positive qualities like tolerance, forgiveness, cheerfulness, concern for others, etc., which are very conducive to a happy married life.

Setting Right Sexual Disharmonies

The major causes for the increase in sexual disharmonies are tension, insecurity and emotional conflicts created by modern life. There are two important factors that determine human sexual behaviour viz., instinctive drives and social influences. Our sex conduct has been predominantly controlled and determined by modern society, which usually results in an emotional conflict between desire and inhibitions. Among primitive people, where social life and sexual standards are simple and natural, sexual inadequacies are not encountered. In our culture, however, the tension of daily living may lead to many disharmonies in the sexual life of a couple.

Yoga stresses physical and mental poise to accelerate **relaxation through reduction of tension and clarity of mind.** Once mental and emotional equanimity is achieved through constant practise of Yoga, sexual disharmonies among married partners would disappear.

Yoga for Impotence

In simple terms, impotence may be defined as the inability to have satisfactory sexual relations with the opposite sex. At times, the terms 'impotence' and 'infertility' are misconstrued. A man may be highly potent but not necessarily fertile. Similarly, a man may be fertile but may not be sexually potent.

The causes for impotence may be due to **constitutional disorders** like hormone deficiency of the sex organs or other constitutional factors that lead to diminution of sexual desire.

There are a number of **psychological factors** too causing impotence in men. In most cases, it is caused by emotional factors like mental conflicts, various fears and anxieties, neurotic tendencies and negative influences in childhood and certain teachings condemning sex as obscene and vulgar. These factors result in an aversion to sex.

Yoga can definitely **remedy impotence** caused by constitutional disorders as well as psychological factors. The practise of certain Asanas would invigorate the functions of various ductless glands, particularly the sex gland, and thereby vigorously activate all organs connected with sex. In this way, constitutional disorders causing impotence are remedied through regular practise of certain Asanas. For details refer to the section on 'Practise of Asanas'.

Similarly, psychological factors causing impotence can also be remedied through the practise of Pranayama and meditation. Pranayama particularly helps tone up the nervous system and thereby ensures mental equilibrium. Similarly, regular practise of meditation tremendously improves emotional stability and ultimately removes psychological factors causing impotence.

There are certain subtle techniques in Yoga that are quite simple to perform but very effective in boosting the sexual urge to a considerable extent. These **techniques are kept highly confidential** by many Yogis in India and are therefore not explained in any of the books on Yoga, nor are they disclosed in public. The Guru passes on these techniques orally to the disciple after ascertaining his sincerity and honesty to ensure he will not misuse the techniques.

Students and Yoga

Present-day students are future citizens of the country. So, a strong nation, both in **intellect and discipline**, has to be moulded from these students.

The aim of education is not mere transmission of ideas and information from one to another. It involves the creation of a full-fledged personality, both in mind and body.

Students have a lot of energy. So, it is the duty of educationists to channel this energy for productive purposes. The main problem faced by students is **controlling their minds** to channelise them for concentrated learning and productive utilisation of energy. Most students are adolescents and there is every chance of their brimming enthusiasm being diverted from the main objective of learning to stray activities. It is here that Yoga can do tremendous good. When students are made to practise certain Yogic Asanas and Pranayama, they get into the habit of a **disciplined system of life**. This leads to the control of body and mind, creates awareness and helps them become responsible citizens. Yoga helps a wandering mind concentrate on a specific task with single-minded devotion. It inculcates a positive approach to life.

Also, if students regularly practise Pranayama, their nervous system gets toned up and **memory, concentration, intelligence and imagination will develop substantially**. Thus, practise of Yoga by students not only helps them control their body, mind and emotions, but also improves mental, emotional and other faculties.

Yoga for Youthfulness

Scientists are curious to know whether **old age can be put off** through deliberate and conscious efforts. They have discovered various factors that promote ageing. In order to "**grow old youthfully**" or gracefully, the elasticity of the body must be maintained. As one ages, hardened mineral substances replace the bone cartilages of childhood. These mineral substances are lime salts and calcium phosphate. When the percentage of these mineral matter increase, the cartilages gradually begin to ossify and become more and more brittle. In advanced years, on reaching an abnormal proportion, the mineral deposits in the bones cause old age.

Old age is also caused due to certain chemical changes in the circulatory system. As the years advance, an accumulation of sedimentary mineral deposits occurs in the circulatory system, leading to **non-elasticity** of the body in general and arteriosclerosis (**hardening of arteries**) in particular. This process hastens old age.

Similarly, as a person advances in age, his muscular tissues harden, leading to stiffness and non-elasticity in the muscular system. Moreover, hardening of muscular tissues results in loss of normal tone and pliancy. These factors ultimately disturb the natural harmony between various internal organs and always end in some form of physical deterioration vaguely called old age.

In order to maintain youthfulness and postpone old age, the natural elasticity, balance and coordination between various parts of the body and the internal organs has to be maintained in perfect condition. The most desirable aspect in maintaining youthfulness is the preservation of a child-like adaptation of every part of the body, which upholds the relative harmony between and within the internal organs.

In his book, *Old Age – Its Causes and Prevention,* Samford Bennet explained the difference between the young and the old in the following words:

"The elasticity of the youth gives place to the non-elasticity of old age. The only difference between a young body and an old one seems to be the elasticity of the former and the non-elasticity of the latter."

Thus, in order to maintain youth and defer old age, one must **develop suppleness of the body**. All the Yogic Asanas are designed to make each and every limb of the body supple and elastic. Moreover, most of the static as well as dynamic Asanas provide a **massaging effect** to all the internal organs and thereby invigorate their functions to the optimum level, which generally brings about sound health in a person and promotes the maintenance of energy and a spirit of youthfulness in the practitioner.

It is now scientifically proved that the whole world is saturated with **electro-magnetic waves,** composed of positive and negative forces. We receive electromagnetically charged cosmic radiations from outer space. Our life itself is a manifestation of the electric current in one form or another expressed in terms of the cellular, cerebral and nervous system operating in the human organism. The human body receives certain subtle **electrical magnetism that travels from the sky to the earth and from the earth to the sky**. Ordinarily, when a person is in an upright position, these waves flow from head to foot, but when the body is inverted, these currents reverse their normal direction in the body.

The harmonious interplay of positive and negative electric currents in the human body is responsible for its good health. Illness or disease of the human body is the result of these currents going out of balance. If these currents are made to change their directions, they can regain equilibrium and, thereby, the physical and mental health of the person is restored. All the **topsy-turvy Asanas** perform this function of making the positive and negative currents in the body operate in harmonious fashion. Therefore, a person consistently practising topsy-turvy Asanas like Sanvanga Asana and Sirsha Asana maintains sound health throughout his life and **postpones the ageing process** for a considerable length of time.

Moreover, the process of ageing and direction of time is associated with the upright position and the normal flow of these currents. When the position of the body is reversed, as when performing topsy-turvy Asanas, the ageing process and **time is also reversed**. In this way, the usual direction of human development is reversed and youthfulness is regained and maintained.

Yoga for Curing Diseases

It has been proved scientifically that practise of Yoga **eliminates chronic and incurable diseases**. The process of cure may be **slow but** the result is **certain** and **permanent**, provided the practitioner meticulously follows the prescribed methods and techniques of Yoga.

Doctors in the field of psychosomatic medicine and psychiatry suggest Yogic therapy to their patients. They have realised that Yoga helps eliminate psychophysical tensions that linger among patients even after their recovery from mental and nervous disorders.

Modern society forces us into **unnatural and artificial ways of living**. We don't eat, drink, sleep, breathe or clothe ourselves properly, resulting in diseases, disorders and ailments. Faulty ways of living, bad habits, improper food, and wrong thinking all give rise to negative emotions such as fear, hatred, prejudice, and despair, causing short term as well as prolonged malfunctioning of the human system.

Since the **root cause** of all diseases are **wrong habits and mistakes** committed by an individual, the **cure lies in correcting them**. The approach of Yogic therapy is therefore based on the principle that diseases can be **cured by the patient's own efforts** – self-control, patience and perseverance. It does not believe in medicines and surgery that are mostly external in nature. It emphasises the practise of Yogic Asanas, Pranayama, meditation and proper diet for curing all types of disease. Under Yogic treatment the **patient has to strive hard himself** for curing his disease without depending on doctors. The Yoga expert who acts as a doctor will inform and, if necessary, demonstrate the methods and techniques of Yoga suitable for the particular disease and it is left to patients to practise them and observe the prescribed diet.

Many **medical men** practising Yoga have expressed their **conviction** that there is something in Yoga that cannot be provided by any other system of medicine.

The approach of **modern medicine**, by and large, is **only to remove symptoms** of the disease temporarily and it rarely attempts removing the root cause of the disease. When a man suffers from headache he is given a pill that quickly relieves the pain. Unfortunately, the pain returns with greater intensity after a few days. This is due to the piecemeal treatment of symptoms and not the disease. For example, asthma, diabetes etc. are not easily amenable to modern medical treatment. A **chronic disease** is **deep-rooted in the organism** of an individual and so symptomatic treatment cannot help to remove it totally but may only provide some relief from pain and discomfort.

On the other hand, **Yogic therapy cures all types of diseases**, including chronic ones, because **it revitalises the entire human system** through the following processes:

1. **Constipation** is one of the root causes for most diseases. Most **Asanas** are designed to remove constipation. Further, the Asanas render the body light and supple, which are indicators of sound health.
2. Hatha Yoga has evolved **six purificatory processes** known as Shat Karma. Their practise ensures purification of the entire system through removal of toxins in the body. For most chronic diseases, **Shat Karma** is advised.

3. **Pranayama revitalises the nervous system** and removes all defects in the **respiratory system**. It also paves the way for toning the **circulatory system**. Most diseases of the respiratory system are cured through Pranayama.
4. **Meditation** brings about **mental poise, emotional balance and a dispassionate outlook** towards life. Worldwide, doctors and scientists have scientifically proved the contribution of meditation in removing physical and psychological stress.

Thus the approach of **Yogic therapy is practical and natural** and the cure is permanent, though the process may sometimes be **slow and time-consuming**.

Generally, the approach of Yoga is **curative as well as preventive**. Regular practise of Yoga ensures sound health throughout life for an individual and also provides insurance against the onslaughts of chronic diseases in the later part of one's life.

A First-hand Experience

I was a **sickly child** with a weak constitution. Indigestion, dyspepsia, asthma, arthritis, stomach pain, headache, fever, etc. were my regular lot. Poor digestion and low energy were a constant problem.

At the **age of 37**, on the recommendation of an allopathic doctor, Dr Dhananjaya, I **began practising** Yogic Asanas, Pranayama, Shat Karma and meditation. Within four to five months my health improved considerably. Thereafter, I took serious interest in Yoga and followed a set regimen and my health **continued to improve** day by day.

I now **advocate Yoga** with religious fervour to all participants of my training programmes for the development of an integrated personality. Now I am in my late sixties, but wake up between 3 and 4 in the morning and continue to work till 11 in the night without an iota of tiredness. My energy levels are very high. **I attribute my superb health to the practise of Yoga.**

Yoga and Religion

Yoga is **not a religion** but just a science expounding certain methods and techniques for **all-round development of the personality**. Therefore, what is required in Yoga is not faith in a particular religion but practise with conviction.

Yoga is very well known as one of the six orthodox systems of Indian philosophy. It was specially evolved by **Hindu saints and monks**. However, it has **nothing to do with any religious doctrines or dogmas**. It is primarily concerned with the practise of some techniques and methods suited to develop the physical, mental and emotional faculties of man. Therefore, it should be **viewed as a Science of Man** dealing with disciplining the body, mind and emotion. It does **not** attempt to advocate the **faith of any particular religion**. There are various branches of science dealing with different aspects of man such as physiology, sociology etc. We do not make any demarcation of these sciences, viz., Hindu physiology, Christian anatomy and Muslim psychology. Similarly, there is **no question of Hindu Yoga or Christian Yoga**.

Unfortunately, some devout Christians, particularly Catholics, are often opposed to the very word 'Yoga', thinking it is one of the doctrines of Hinduism. They are apprehensive that the practise of Yoga is against Christian faith. In his book *Christian Yoga*, Rev. Fr. J.M. Dechanet, O.S.B., a veteran Catholic priest, explained how the techniques of Yoga would enhance Christian life to a considerable extent. He said: ***"Every day the exercises, and indeed the whole ascetic discipline of Yoga, make it easier for the grace of Christ to flow in me. I feel my hunger for God growing and my thirst for righteousness, and my desire to be a Christian in the full strength of the word – to be for Christ, to be of Christ, without any half-measures or reservations... There shall be no compromise; but only borrowing of methods to be adopted immediately and introduced into an ascetic discipline authentically Christian in tenor and spirit."***

He further narrated his initial experiences with Yoga in the following words: ***"What I then read about Yoga and about some of its aims simply encouraged me to embark on, and then go through with, an experiment about the appropriateness of which I became convinced at the very first attempt. Yoga, I found, was first of all a particular way of fashioning oneself, the way of the man who by means of certain disciplines, both physiological (postures and breath-control) and psychical (focussing of thought), was joined; that is to say, in a condition of coherence in accordance with vital functions, and in a state of balance such that life could be controlled and made effective. This is therefore the opposite of fragmented living, of naïve incoherence, impotence and unawareness... On the physical plane, the problems of general health disappeared; I no longer suffered from those fits of tiredness and temperature that pointed clearly to overwork. I found myself possessed of an extremely supple body, ready to serve me and the life of the spirit..."***

After the publication of this book, the outlook of the Christian community underwent a thorough change regarding Yoga. Many Catholic priests and nuns started showing keen interest in Yoga. I had several opportunities to conduct Yoga courses exclusively for these people all over the world.

My personal experience is almost identical with that of Fr. Dechanet. Consistent practise of Yoga has brought tremendous improvement in my health, as mentioned earlier. Considerable change has also occurred in my behavioural pattern. A calm and serene feeling has set within me permanently and I do not feel inclined to even get angry with anybody for anything. I certainly feel that it is possible for me to love my enemies. And I sincerely feel that regular practise of **Yoga has enabled me to lead a better Christian life**. All sincere and regular practitioners of Yoga can have the same experience.

Yoga and Vegetarianism

It may be observed that many Yogis in India staunchly advocate that practitioners take only vegetarian food. Yogis consider wilful adoption of a vegetarian diet implies a moral act that strengthens control over oneself in the first instance and then over one's environment. This need for **exercising self-control** arises only in the case of born non-vegetarians and not for born vegetarians. Hence it facilitates vegetarians practising Yoga without exercising any self-control, whereas many non-vegetarians feel hesitant to practise Yoga as long as they continue to eat non-vegetarian food.

In the past, vegetarianism evolved as an Indian philosophy based purely on the **principle of Ahimsa**, which is one of the tenets of Raja Yoga. Thus, vegetarianism becomes not a mere dietetic principle but a religious doctrine.

Here, the words of **Swami Vivekananda**, a noted exponent of Yoga, are worth quoting:

"The test of Ahimsa is absence of jealousy. Any man may do a good deed or make a good gift on the spur of the moment, or under the pressure of some superstition or priest craft, but the real lover of mankind is he who is jealous of none. The so-called great man of the world may all be seen to become jealous of each other for a small name, for a little fame and for a few bits of gold. So long as this jealousy exists in a heart, it is far away from the perfection of Ahimsa. The cow does not eat meat nor does the sheep. Are they great Yogis, great non-injurers (Ahimsakas)? Any fool may abstain from eating this or that; surely that gives him no more distinction than to herbivorous animals. The man who will mercilessly cheat widows and orphans, and do the vilest deeds for money is worse than any brute even if he lives entirely on grass. The man whose heart never cherishes even the thought of injury to anyone, who rejoices at the prosperity of even his greatest enemy, that man is the Bhakta, he is the Yogi, he is the Guru of all, even though he lives every day of his life on the flesh of swine. Therefore, we must always remember that external practices have value only as it helps to develop internal purity. It is better to have internal purity alone, when attention to external observances is not practicable. But woe unto the man and woe unto the nation that forgets the real, internal, spiritual essentials of religion and mechanically clutches with death-like grasp at all external forms and never lets them go. The forms have value only so far as they are expressions of the life within. If they have ceased to express life, crush them out without mercy."

(*Bhakti Yoga*, pp. 59-60.)

From the above words of Swami Vivekananda, we may now understand that vegetarianism is only an external practice, which does not have much relevance to the real practise of Yoga.

Many non-vegetarians are hesitant to practise Yoga believing that non-vegetarian diet coupled with the practise of Yoga would harm their health. There is no scientific evidence to prove this. The practitioner of Yoga is always advised to be moderate in everything. The ***Bhagavad Gita*** states:

"Yoga is not possible for him who eats too much or for him who abstains too much from eating; it is not for him who sleeps too much or too little. For him who is moderate in eating and recreation, temperate in his actions, who is regulated in sleep and wakefulness."

Therefore, it is not the type of food that one takes but the manner and attitude with which it is taken that is of paramount importance. However, it may be stressed that the practitioner of Yoga should always have **proper control over food habits**. Do also remember that we **eat to live and not live to eat**.

Guidance from the Guru

There cannot be two opinions regarding the preferability of having a competent Guru (teacher) to teach Yoga. It is always advantageous and beneficial to attend classes in schools or colleges to learn any art or science than to undertake self-study through books or correspondence.

Even though the benefits of Yoga are widely acknowledged, competent teachers are unfortunately not available in required numbers. However, if a proper Guru is not available, a person sincerely interested in learning Yoga may try to initiate the practice by referring to some standard books on Yoga. Initially, he may start with very simple Asanas and only when he wants to learn advanced techniques would he require the guidance of a competent Guru.

It is not good to remain passive just because a Guru is not available to teach Yoga. If a person is very earnest in his approach he will definitely find a suitable Guru. Therefore, one **need not wait for a Guru** to take up Yoga. In this context, Swami Sivananda's words are worth quoting:

"Do not hesitate. Do not wait to get a Guru who will sit by your side and watch you daily... If you are sincere, regular and systematic and if you follow the rules and instructions of this book very carefully, there will not be trouble at all. You will get success. Slight errors may crop up in the beginning, but it does not matter. Do not unnecessarily be alarmed. Do not give up the practices. You will learn how to adjust. Common sense, instinct, the still inner voice of the soul will help you on the path. Everything will come out smoothly in the end. Start the practice this very second in right earnest and become a real Yogi."

(*The Science of Pranayama*, the Yoga-Vedanta Forest Academy, 1962, pp. 105.)

Yoga and the Elderly

Authorities on Yoga have different views on this aspect. Some say that Yoga should be taken up only after the age of nine and others advocate that even children above the age of three can practise simple Yogic Asanas.

The real problem arises only with **elderly persons** after the age of 40. As a person grows older, his body stiffens and flexibility of the limbs decreases. Hence, an elderly person taking up Yoga finds it difficult to perform certain Asanas well. However, they may attempt to **practise simple Asanas** without making any strong and jerky movements. Over some time, they may be able to attain flexibility and suppleness of body.

Yoga is not confined only to Yoga Asanas. The practices include Pranayama, Mudras, Bhandas, Shat Karmas and meditation. Elderly persons who cannot perform Yogic Asanas can very well take up **Pranayama and Meditation.** There is absolutely no age restriction for anybody to take up Yoga. But the practise should be continuous and there is no need to stop it at any age. As long as a person is capable of performing the Asanas comfortably, he can go ahead.

However, as a person advances beyond 60 years, he may restrict his time for practising Asanas and devote more time for Pranayama and meditation. I have seen many elderly persons even beyond the age of 70 performing some of the difficult Asanas with ease. This depends upon regular practise over a long period.

The Best Time to Practise

In order to derive maximum benefit, Yoga should be practised early in the morning before sunrise. One should develop the habit of waking up at least before 5 A.M. Since the mind is fresh in the morning, meditation can be taken up first. Then Asanas, Pranayama, Mudras and Bhandas could follow.

Usually, the limbs are stiff in the morning. So, it is difficult to perform advanced Asanas. These can be performed with ease and comfort in the evening. The stress and strain of the day can be removed if Asanas and Pranayama are done in the evening.

The Best Place to Practise

Yoga should be practised in a **well-ventilated, clean and airy room**, free from insects and noise. The floor of the room must be even. The room should be spacious enough for free movement of all limbs. Greater benefits could be derived if Yoga is practised on the **sands of rivers**, in open places or by the **seaside**.

Cold Water Bath and Yoga

Most people practising Yoga prefer to take bath in cold water. A **cold water bath invigorates the nervous system** and promotes effective blood circulation. However, it is **not necessary** to take a bath in cold water. When the weather is cold, it is better to take bath in warm water. This can be varied according to **individual requirements**.

I take bath in cold water. When the weather is very cold, I then take bath in warm water. I practise Yoga after bath. The body gains flexibility after bath and Yoga should be practised preferably after bath. Taking bath both before and after doing Yoga refreshes the body and mind.

Smoking, Drinking and Yoga

Many people are under the impression that Yoga is something mysterious and supernatural, therefore, certain habits like smoking and drinking should be avoided before taking up Yoga. A person may feel it is better not to practise Yoga rather than to stop smoking or drinking in order to take up Yoga. Advising a person to do so is not required. It is akin to advising a person to learn swimming first before plunging into the water.

My simple suggestion to all those who are addicted to smoking or drinking is that they **need not worry about their habits, but simply start practising Yoga** in a milder form to begin with. In course of time they will gain better health, steadiness of mind, self-control over themselves and achieve emotional balance and, soon, it will not be surprising if they give up these habits effortlessly.

Regularity

There is no scientific evidence that Yoga has harmful effects if it is stopped abruptly. In order to derive complete and full benefits from Yoga, one should be **regular and consistent** in the practice. Many start with enthusiasm but stop later. Such persons do not suffer any harmful effects at all, but they do not derive the full benefits of Yoga.

Part Two

Theory and Practise of Asanas

Yogic Asanas and Physical Exercises

Physical exercises help **develop the muscles** through mechanical movement, whereas Yogic Asanas cater to the development of **both the body and mind**. Through constant practise of Yoga one can even have control over involuntary muscles of the body.

Physical exercises are done through **fast movement of the muscles**, whereas Yogic Asanas should be performed with **ease and comfort** and all undue strain and exertion of the body must be scrupulously avoided.

Physical exercises do **not guarantee a healthy body**. The practise of Yogic Asanas ensures a healthy body, which is a state when all the organs of the body function perfectly under **intelligent control of the mind**.

The **heart** is put to tremendous **strain** during the performance of physical exercises, as they involve rapid movement of the muscles. In the practise of Yogic Asanas all movements are slow and gradual with proper breathing and relaxation. This **revitalises the heart** and does not produce any type of strain.

The main objective of physical exercise is to **increase blood circulation** and also improve the capacity for intake of oxygen through rapid movement of the muscles and other parts of the body. This can be easily achieved via the practise of Asanas through simple movement of the spine and various joints of the body with **deep breathing** and without any violent movement of any kind.

One of the most glaring differences between physical exercises and Yogic Asanas is that after the completion of a course of physical exercises one is completely **exhausted and tired**. On the other hand, the performance of Asanas is done slowly and gradually through rhythmic movement of the body synchronised with the breath. Our forefathers so ingeniously designed the Asanas that while performing the Asanas **energy is generated within the body** and, therefore, after completion of a series of Yogic Asanas one feels **refreshed and energetic**. There is no question of fatigue or tiredness after the completion of Yogic Asanas. While performing the Asanas, various limbs of the body are stretched and maintained for a particular duration and then they are released slowly and gracefully. This process of stretching and releasing in a rhythmic manner brings about a wonderful relaxation in the entire body.

Yogic Asanas are meant to **tone up the internal organs** of the body and to revitalise the working of the **endocrine glands**. On the other hand, physical exercises are meant to build muscles of the body. Yogic Asanas ensure **better health**, whereas physical exercises provide good physique. However, Yogic Asanas and physical exercises can be practised simultaneously. The only condition required for the performance of physical exercises is that they should be done after ensuring a break of half an hour on completion of Yogic Asanas. Both should not be continuously practised.

The best way of combining these two aspects is that in the **morning Yogic Asanas** could be performed and in the **evening physical exercises** may be done.

Time Limit for Asanas

There is no time limit for individual Asanas and this is left completely to the convenience of the practitioner. There are two types of Asanas; one is **static** and the other **dynamic**. The dynamic Asanas could be repeated a number of times. This can be done without getting tired. As far as the static Asanas are concerned, the practitioner is expected to be in a posture for a prescribed time. There is **no stipulated time** for individual Asanas. However, if the practitioner feels some **pain** in any part of the body while performing the Asanas, he should immediately **stop**.

The time devoted for the individual Asana should be of short duration in the initial stage and this duration should be gradually increased on the basis of the comfort and ease with which a person can perform. The time at the disposal of the practitioner and the objective for which he is practising are the prime determining factors.

Closed or Open Eyes

In the **early stages** of the practise of Asanas, it is better to **open the eyes**, which will enable one to observe whether they are being done perfectly. If the postures are wrong they can be checked and corrected. One can keep the eyes closed only when the performance of a particular Asana is proper and satisfactory. When the **eyes are closed**, the mind becomes calm and one can look inward and concentrate mainly on the **benefits of the Asana**.

Perfection of Performance

Many wish to know how to find out whether a person is performing the Asanas correctly. One of the important factors to be remembered in the practise of Yogic Asanas is that it should be done in a gradual manner. Nobody should attempt to master all the Asanas quickly. Therefore, caution is to be exercised to ensure that **no pain or discomfort** develops in any part of the body. If discomfort is felt while performing an Asana, it may be presumed that the particular Asana was not performed properly. This is an indication to stop the performance of that Asana immediately and switch over to another.

Sequence of Asanas

The Asanas should be practised in perfect sequence or the practitioner will not derive maximum benefit. The **sequence should be meticulously observed**, particularly in the **initial stages**.

The order in which the Asanas must be performed depends upon the **number of Asanas** chosen and the **time at the disposal** of the practitioner. However, certain general principles can be evolved to formulate the sequence of doing the Asanas. **After** completing a **forward bending** Asana it is better to immediately do a **backward bending** one to act as a counter-posture. This is the main reason why it is generally recommended that Matsya Asana should always be performed immediately after completing Sarvanga Asana. Similarly, Chakra Asana may be done after Hal Asana.

Strict adherence to the sequence may be followed in the initial stage. Once mastery is obtained in the performance of the Asanas, one can create one's own sequence on the basis of personal requirements.

Synchronisation of Breath

The **breath** should be **properly synchronised** while performing the Asanas depending upon the manner in which the body is positioned. One of the essential features that distinguish Yogic Asanas from physical exercises is that greater emphasis is placed on the synchronisation of the breath.

While explaining the practical aspects of the individual Asanas in the subsequent pages, specific mention has been made about how the breath must be synchronised.

Points to Ponder

1. Asanas should be performed in a **slow and graceful** manner without any jerky or violent movements.
2. **Breaths** should be properly **synchronised** with the movement of various parts of the body.
3. The **mind** should be **calm** and **relaxed**, saturated in sublime and serene thoughts. All negative feelings like envy, jealousy, malice, anger, and hatred should be scrupulously avoided.
4. Asanas should not be practised in a mechanical way but must be considered a purposeful activity. One should **mentally repeat** that by doing a particular Asana he would derive certain **benefits**. Specific mention has been made in the subsequent pages regarding the aspects on which one should **utilise autosuggestion** while doing the Asana. This is mentioned for every Asana under the subtitle **Activate the Subconscious Mind**.
5. **After completion** of every posture, **relax** the entire body by lying down in Shava Asana for a few seconds and then take up the practise of the next Asana.
6. **A set of Asanas** should be selected and practised regularly in proper sequence.

PRACTISE OF ASANAS

Asana No. 1

SURYA NAMASKAR

(*Sulutation to the Sun Posture*)

Special Remarks

If there is not much time to practise Asanas, Pranayama and meditation, Surya Namaskar alone can ensure the benefits of all types of Yogic practices.

Surya Namaskar combines the benefits of physical exercise, Asanas and Pranayama. It is a multi-stage Asana. Being a combination of 12 Asanas, one can gain the benefits of all the Asanas involved in it.

In this Asana there are 12 spinal positions. The vertebral column is bent forward and backward alternately with deep breathing. There is contraction on the abdomen and diaphragm when the body is bent forward. When the body bends backward the chest expands and deep breathing occurs automatically. In this way, flexibility increases and breathing is corrected.

This Asana is done preferably in the morning while facing the rising sun. If you are unable to watch the rising sun for one reason or the other, practise Surya Namaskar facing the East. Start doing it thrice only and gradually increase the number.

Technique

Position One – *Pranama Asana* (Prayer Posture)

- Stand erect facing the East, with hands relaxed by the sides.
- Inhale and join the palms in Namaskara Mudra on the chest. **(Picture 1)**
- Breathe normally and concentrate on the rising sun.

Position Two – *Hasta Uttan Asana* (Raised Arms Posture)

- Inhale and raise the arms high.
- Bend backward as far as possible
- Hold the breath in. **(Picture 2)**

Position Three – *Pada Hasta Asana* (Head to Foot Posture)

- Without bending the knees, bend forward while exhaling till the palms touch the floor.
- Stay in this posture as long as you feel comfortable. **(Picture 3)**

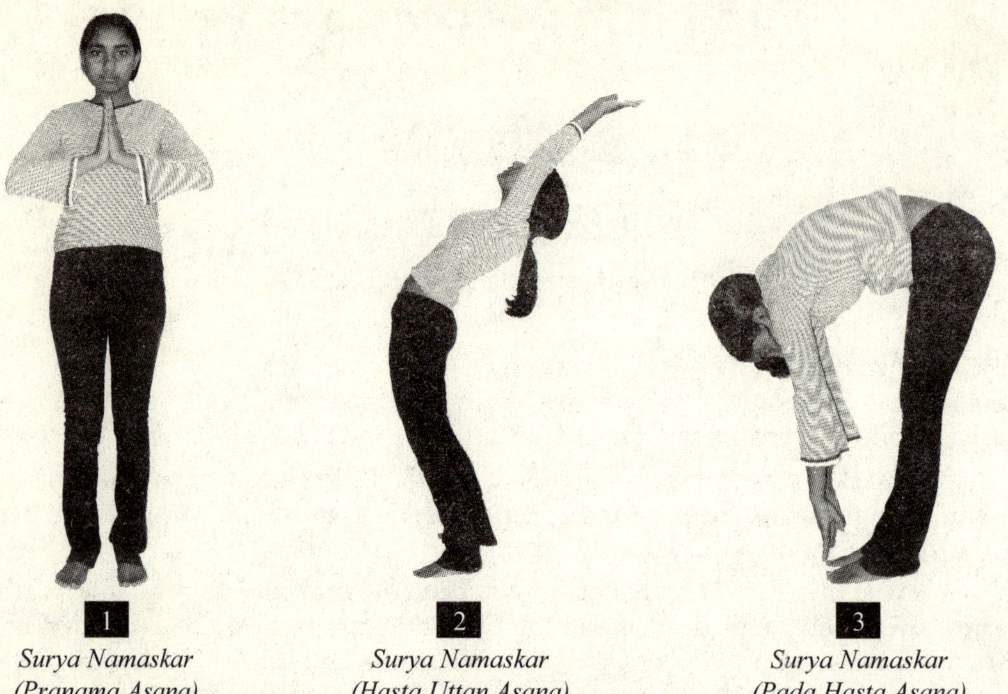

1 Surya Namaskar (Pranama Asana)

2 Surya Namaskar (Hasta Uttan Asana)

3 Surya Namaskar (Pada Hasta Asana)

Position Four – *Ashwasanchalana Asana* (Equestrian Posture)

- Without inhaling, bend the left knee and stretch the left leg as far back as possible until the palms rest on the floor.
- The weight of the body should now be supported on the two hands, the left foot, the right knee and the right toes. Hold your breath. **(Picture 4)**

Position Five – *Parvat Asana* (Mountain Posture)

- Exhale as you straighten the left leg to place the left foot beside the right one.
- Raise the buttocks and keep the head up, with the heels touching the floor.
- The body should form two sides of a triangle with the legs and arms unbent. **(Picture 5)**

Position Six – *Ashtanga Namaskar Asana* (Salute with Total Surrender Posture)

- Lower the body to the floor so that the toes of the feet, the knees, the chest, the hands and the chin touch the floor.
- The hips and the abdomen should be raised.
- Do not breathe. **(Picture 6)**

Position Seven – *Bhujanga Asana* (Cobra Posture)

- While inhaling, raise the body from the waist up by straightening the arms.

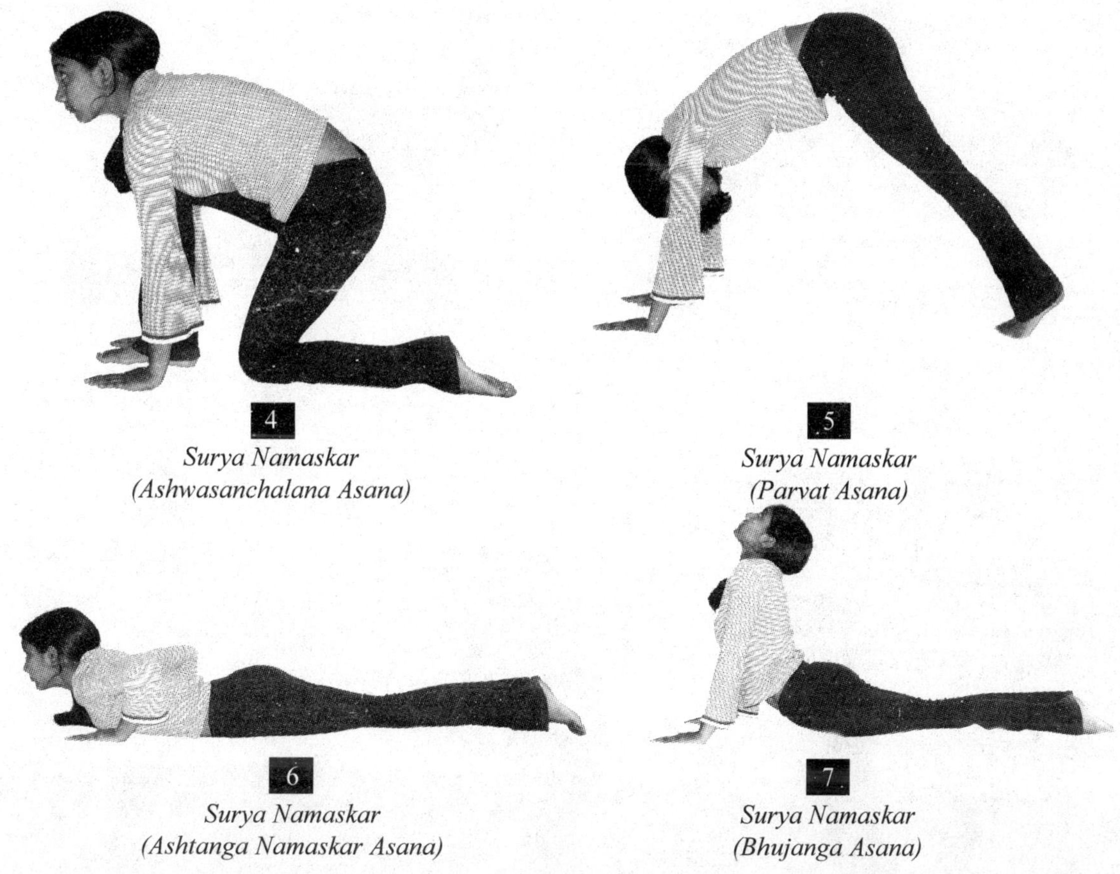

4
Surya Namaskar
(Ashwasanchalana Asana)

5
Surya Namaskar
(Parvat Asana)

6
Surya Namaskar
(Ashtanga Namaskar Asana)

7
Surya Namaskar
(Bhujanga Asana)

- Bend as far back as possible. The spine should be bent to the maximum. **(Picture 7)**

Position Eight – *Parvat Asana*

This is a repetition of position five.

- Exhale and lift the body.
- Keep the feet and heels flat on the floor. **(Picture 8)**

Position Nine – *Ashwasanchalana Asana*

- This posture corresponds to position four with the legs in alternate positions.
- Inhale and bring the right foot in line with the hands. The left foot and knee should touch the floor.
- Look slightly up. **(Picture 9)**

Position Ten – *Pada Hasta Asana*

- Exhale and bring the left leg forward. Keep the knees straight.
- Bring the head to the third position. **(Picture 10)**

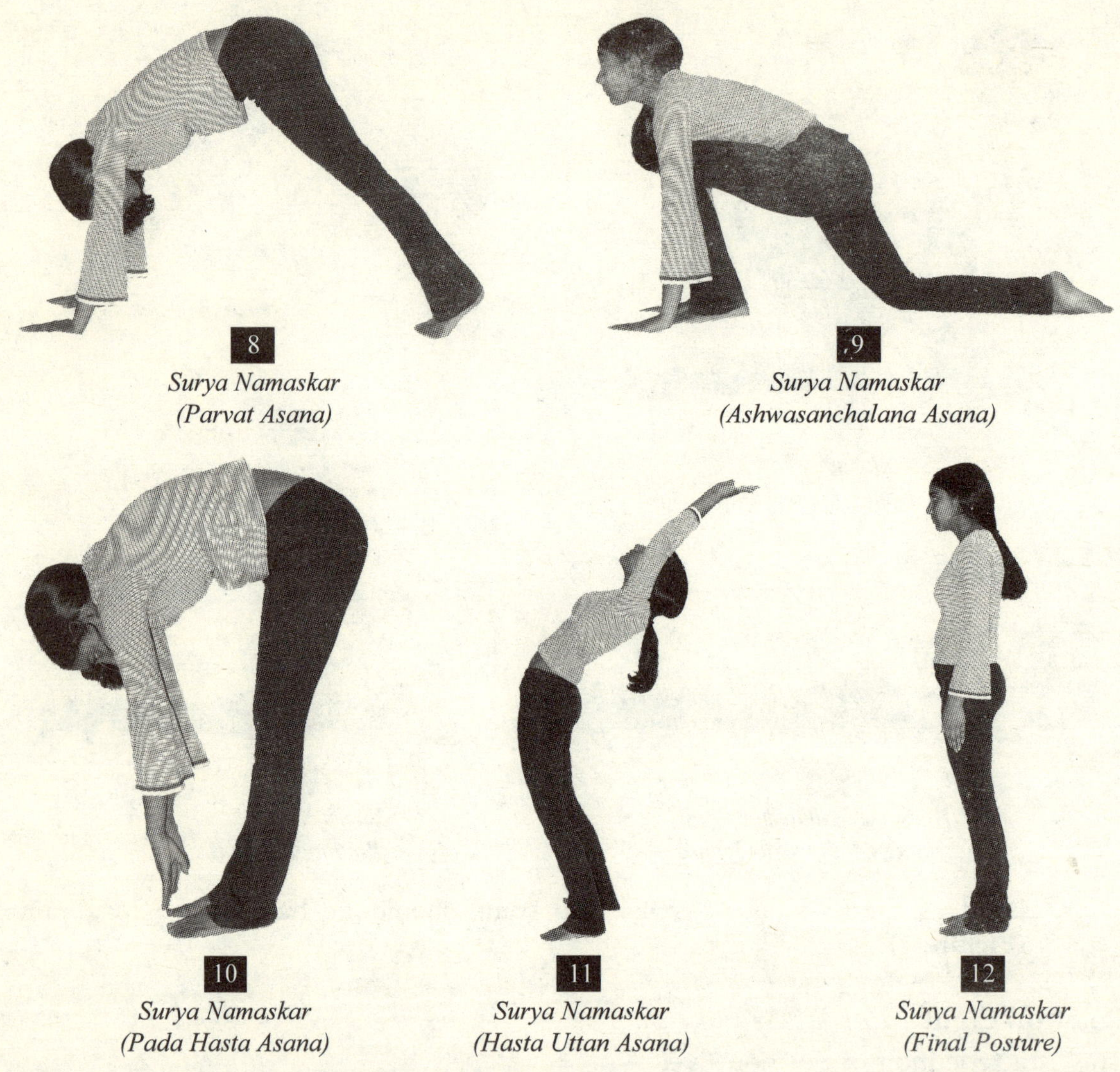

8
Surya Namaskar
(Parvat Asana)

9
Surya Namaskar
(Ashwasanchalana Asana)

10
Surya Namaskar
(Pada Hasta Asana)

11
Surya Namaskar
(Hasta Uttan Asana)

12
Surya Namaskar
(Final Posture)

Position Eleven – *Hasta Uttan Asana*

This is a repetition of position two. **(Picture 11)**

Position Twelve – Final Posture

- Exhale. Drop the arms and relax. **(Picture 12)**

Synchronisation of Breath

Mentioned clearly at every step of doing this Asana.

Benefits

- ❑ Ensures remarkable lightness of body, buoyancy of mind and general feeling of youthfulness.

- Strengthens the neck, arms, back, shoulders, thighs, knees, waist, calves and ankles.
- Exercises the legs and arms mildly, thereby increasing blood circulation.
- Cures kidney trouble by strengthening the back.
- Activates sluggish glands.
- Increases chest size and decreases abdominal girth.
- Retards obesity.
- Boosts blood supply to the entire spinal area and thereby strengthens the heart, lungs, liver, stomach, kidneys and bowels.
- Improves and develops the bust in women and gets rid of menstrual disorders; renders childbearing less painful and improves the quantity and quality of milk in nursing mothers.

Activate the Subconscious Mind

Since it is an excellent Asana for general improvement of health and longevity one may make the following suggestion to oneself while performing this Asana:

"My general health is improving considerably in every respect by doing this Asana."

Suitability

Suitable for all, particularly women, who can derive considerable benefit from this Asana.

Precautions

This Asana is to be performed at the time of the rising sun to derive maximum benefits. After performing this Asana it is necessary to relax by doing Shava Asana. **(Picture 13)** For explanation refer to Asana No. 13.

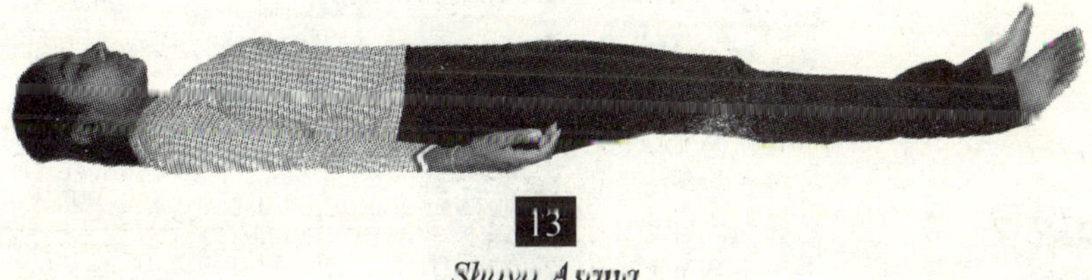

13

Shava Asana

Asana No. 2

SIRSHA ASANA

(*The Headstand Posture*)

Technique

- Assume the position of Vajra Asana. (Refer to **Picture 40**)
- Bring the head down and place it on the ground.
- Interlock the hands and keep them on the backside of your head. (Preparatory Posture: **Picture 14**)
- Slowly raise your legs together and stretch them straight on the ground as much as possible. (Second Posture: **Picture 15**)
- This is a preparatory posture for Sirsha Asana.
- The distance between the elbows should be equal to the distance between the head and elbow of each arm.
- Palms should support the back portion of the head.
- Hands should not support the weight of the body throughout the Asana.
- After assuming the preparatory position slowly bend the knees and raise them upwards.
- The weight of the body is borne by the head supported by the interlocked hands behind and the forearms in the front.
- In the final posture the body should be perfectly straight and exactly vertical. (Final Posture: **Picture 16**)

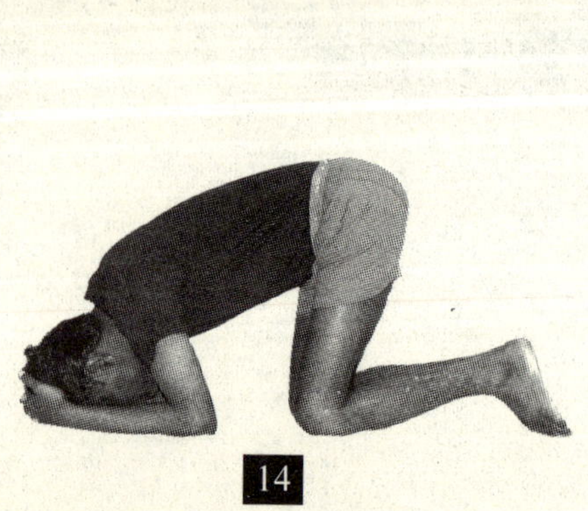

14
Sirsha Asana
(Preparatory Posture)

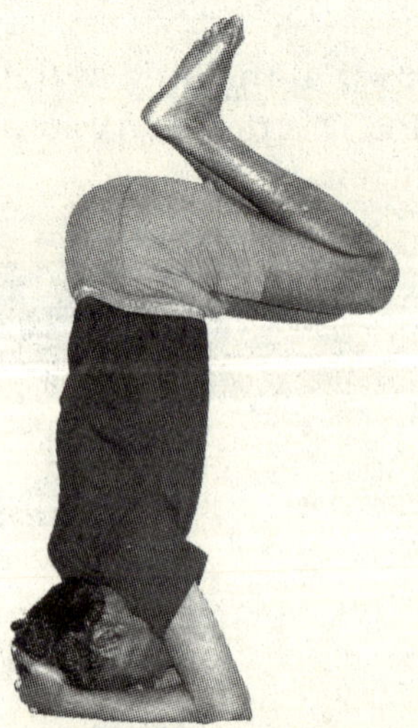

15
Sirsha Asana
(Second Posture)

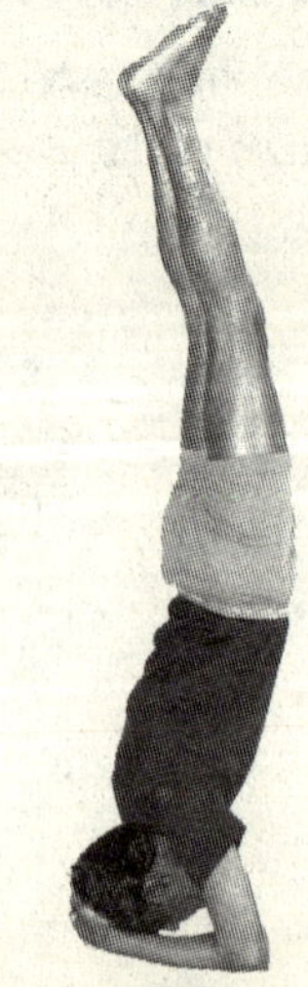

16
Sirsha Asana
(Final Posture)

- The most important point to be remembered in the final posture is that neither the forehead nor the back of the head should rest on the ground but only the crown of the head.
- In the initial stages, beginners should try to do this Asana with the help of a friend. In the absence of anybody, practise this Asana against the corner of a wall so as to prevent falling down.
- The duration of stay in the final posture differs from person to person, depending upon experience and the purpose for which Yogic practices are being undertaken.
- Beginners may stay in the final posture for about 15 to 30 seconds.
- The duration may be extended gradually.
- While raising the body or staying in the final posture the eyes should never become bloodshot. If they do, the posture is presumed to be faulty.
- An advanced way of doing this Asana is to bring both the legs down and form the Padma Asana. This is called Padma Sirsha Asana. (**Picture 17**)

Synchronisation of Breath

Breathe in while lifting the legs up. Maintain normal breathing in the final posture.

How to End

The termination of Sirsha Asana must be slow and gentle. Both legs should be brought down simultaneously with the Padma Asana posture. (**Picture 18**)

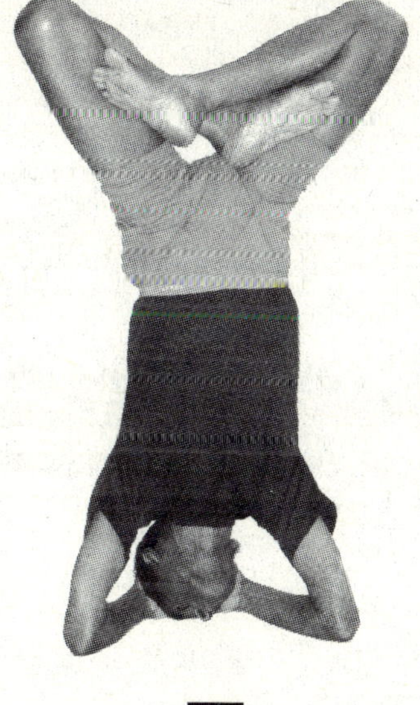

17
Padma Sirsha Asana

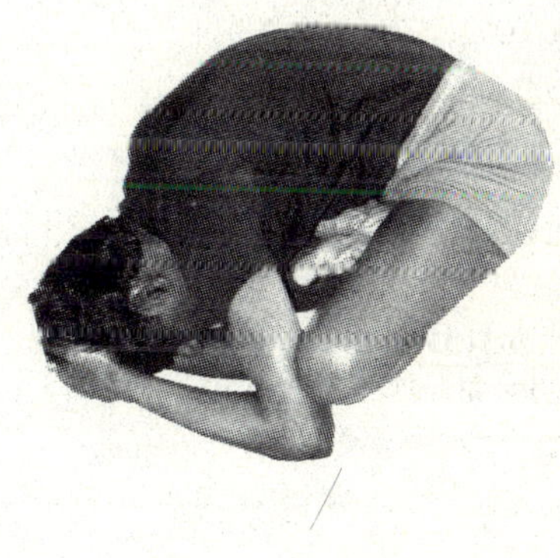

18
Sirsha Asana (Termination)

On termination of this posture, maintain the kneeling position with the head on the floor for at least 30 seconds.

As a sort of counter-pose of this Asana, do Tada Asana for five rounds. This is performed as follows:

TADA ASANA

- Stand erect, interlocking the hands.
- Inhale deeply and simultaneously raise both the heels and the interlocked hands.
- Be in the posture with inner retention for a few seconds. (**Picture 19**)
- Then bring down the raised heels and your hands. Exhale. This is one round of Tada Asana.

This is to be done to ensure proper functioning of the body, particularly blood circulation, which should readjust to normal conditions.

After completing Tada Asana, do Shava Asana without fail. (**Picture 13**)

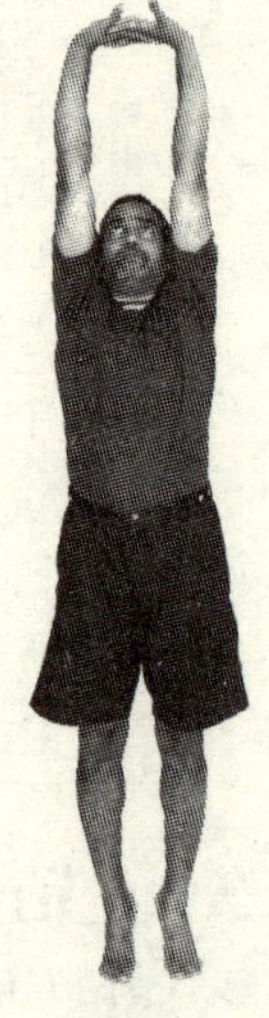

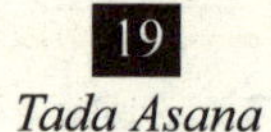

19

Tada Asana

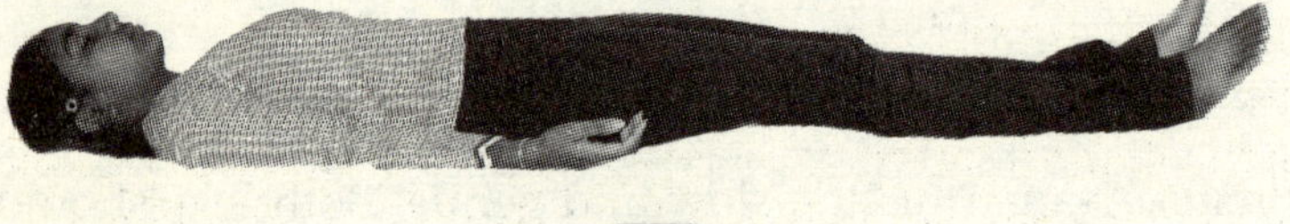

13

Shava Asana

Benefits

- By the action of gravity, the brain receives a richer supply of blood at a somewhat increased pressure. This results in dilation of capillaries and also opens capillaries that are blocked.
- Due to increased amount of blood to the brain, the brain cells are abundantly nourished and rejuvenated.
- Because of the strong flushing action of the blood, the accumulated toxins and waste material are also effectively removed from the brain. This assists in the break-up of cholesterol deposits, which tend to build up on the linings of blood vessels. These deposits are closely related to the occurrence of a blood clot (coronary thrombosis).
- Improves and maintains good physical and mental health.
- Affects the body's entire psycho-physiological mechanism. Produces an immediate and powerful sedation of the nervous system.
- Psychic powers like clairvoyance, telepathy etc. are developed if this Asana is performed for a long duration over a considerable number of years.

- Stagnant or sluggish blood in the abdomen, lungs, and sexual organs is replaced by a good flow of purified blood, which thereby eliminates fatigue caused in these areas.
- Functions of the liver and other digestive organs are activated by decongestion, which thereby improves digestive powers through increased blood supply.
- Urinary problems are eliminated as the kidneys and large intestine are decongested and receive an enhanced blood supply.
- As one grows older, the sex glands are liable to accumulate stagnant blood that brings about loss in functional efficiency. Consistent practise of this Asana activates the sex glands and improves performance of sexual activities.
- Increases blood flow to the eyes and ears and improves their functioning.
- Minor facial wrinkles are eliminated, thereby enabling one to maintain a youthful look.
- Regular practise of this Asana over a long period averts the appearance of grey hair.
- Downward displacement of abdominal organs (visceroptosis) is adjusted, as there is an upward movement of the diaphragm during this Asana. Abdominal organs like the stomach, kidneys, spleen, pancreas, liver etc. are massaged.
- Ensures tranquillity and serenity of mind.
- Cures psychosomatic diseases.
- Cures other diseases like headache, mild asthma, bad hearing, constipation, dyspepsia, enlarged liver, varicose veins, prolapses of sexual organs, diabetes, arthritis etc.
- Female problems during menstruation and menopause and some sexual disorders are remedied.
- Persons suffering from insomnia, defective memory and loss of vitality can derive maximum benefit from this Asana. They will become fountains of energy.
- Provides resistance power to the lungs for any climatic conditions.
- The practitioner is practically relieved from cold, coughs, tonsillitis and bad breath.
- Keeps the body warm.
- Improves haemoglobin content of the blood.
- A regular practitioner gains balance of mind, acquires a sense of self-reliance and improves courage to face untoward situations in life.
- Makes the neck, abdominal walls and thighs powerful. The chest is fully expanded.
- Revitalises all bodily systems by increasing blood flow to the brain and pituitary gland, which is responsible for rectifying many forms of nervous and glandular disorders.
- One of the best Asanas to sublimate sexual energies and help awaken Kundalini Shakti.

Activate the Subconscious Mind

This Asana is considered the King of all Asanas and this is amply proved from the innumerable benefits it confers on the practitioner.

Since this has tremendous therapeutic effects to cure several diseases, patients can conveniently practise this Asana to cure their diseases. They should suggest to themselves as follows while in the final posture:

"I am being cured of my disease."

This is one of the best Asanas to improve memory and intelligence. Therefore, youngsters may use this autosuggestion:

"This Asana improves my memory and intelligence."

In the same manner, the principle of activating the subconscious mind could be applied on the basis of the needs of the individual practitioner.

Precautions

This Asana has to be performed very carefully; otherwise, the practitioner may fall and hurt his body. This should never be attempted without the proper guidance of an expert.

Persons suffering from high blood pressure and heart ailments should not perform this Asana.

Asana No. 3

SARVANGA ASANA

(The Shoulder Stand Posture)

Technique

- Assume a lying down position on the seat with the back to the ground.
- Slowly raise the legs with slow, gradual and constant inhalation. (Preparatory Posture – **Picture 20**)
- The legs must be in a straight line with the trunk and the hips.
- Support the back on the sides with your hands.
- Start exhaling and raise legs upwards towards the sky.
- The trunks and legs should extend straight upwards with the neck forming a right angle, the chest pressing against the chin. (Final Posture – **Picture 21**)
- Avoid jerking and do this Asana very gracefully.
- The whole weight of the body should be thrown on the shoulders.
- Remain in this posture for as long as possible, breathing normally.
- As in Sirsha Asana, you may do Padma Sarvanga Asana. (**Picture 22**)
- After this, exhale and gradually bring down your legs. Release the hands, lie flat and relax.

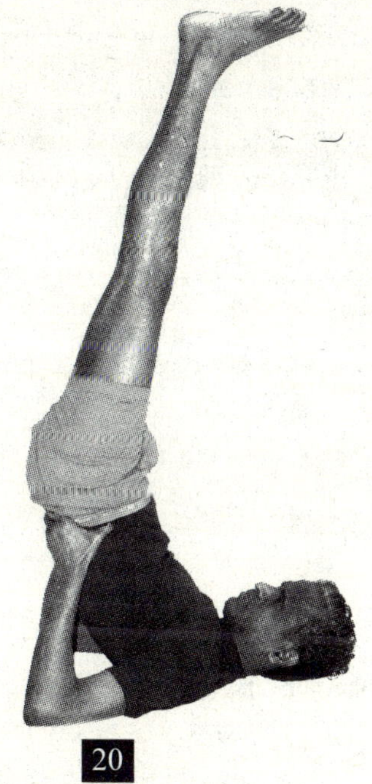

20

Sarvanga Asana (Preparatory Posture)

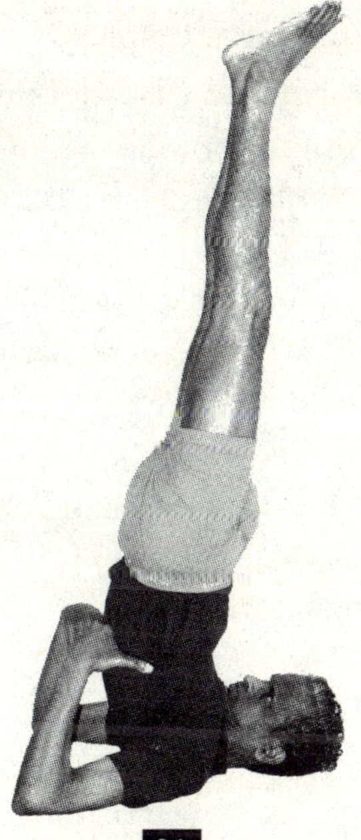

21

Sarvanga Asana (Final Posture)

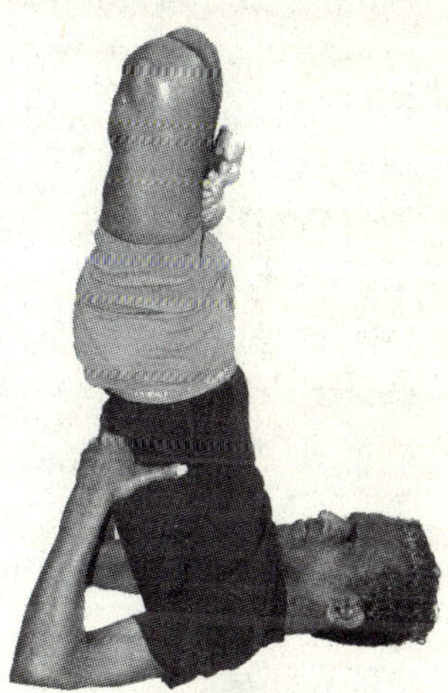

22

Padma Sarvanga Asana

Synchronisation of Breath

As explained in the above example.

Benefits

- ❑ Improves flow of blood to the brain.
- ❑ Stimulates the thyroid gland and keeps it in healthy condition, which results in healthy functioning of all organs of the body.
- ❑ Tones up the nervous and reproductive systems.
- ❑ Adjusts improper body growth.
- ❑ Brings relief from congestion in the abdominal and pelvic regions.
- ❑ Helps cure ailments like constipation, dyspepsia, headache, etc.
- ❑ Keeps the vertebral column in an elastic and pliable condition.
- ❑ Averts calcification of body parts and thereby youth is preserved for longer time.
- ❑ Improves functioning of chords and thereby improves the voice of singers.
- ❑ Aids in awakening Kundalini Shakti.
- ❑ All parts of the body are exercised, energised and activated.
- ❑ Removes respiratory defects in the lungs through internal activation.
- ❑ Gives asthma patients relief.
- ❑ Energises all sex glands and thereby improves sexual activity in both males and females.
- ❑ Ensures great relief from functional disorders of the eyes, ears, nose and throat.
- ❑ Cures appendicitis, gastrointestinal disorders and varicose veins.
- ❑ The face receives extra supply of blood, especially over the forehead and the scalp and thereby helps prevent lines and wrinkles in the face. This preserves the youthful look in both men and women.
- ❑ This Asana has medicinal value for curing impotence, frigidity, lack of sexual power and various other defects of the sexual organs.
- ❑ The heart gets rest as long as you remain in this Asana. This insures one against all heart troubles.
- ❑ For women, this Asana banishes the ever-present menace of irritation and catarrh of the uterus.
- ❑ Improves mental faculty considerably.

Activate the Subconscious Mind

This is one of the best Asanas conferring many benefits on practitioners. However, this is particularly designed to stimulate the thyroid gland and activate the vocal chords.

Since the thyroid gland is responsible for healthy functioning of all organs in the body, it is possible to maintain perfect health throughout one's life by consistent practise of this Asana. Therefore, while doing this Asana, one may suggest the following to activate the subconscious mind:

"My general health is improving to a great extent by doing this Asana."

As this Asana also activates the functioning of the vocal chords, orators, teachers and singers may suggest that their voice has improved considerably by doing this Asana.

Suitability

Suitable for all practitioners.

Precautions

This Asana should not be attempted by persons suffering from high blood pressure, heart ailments, enlarged thyroid, liver or spleen problems.

The Importance

This is a good substitute for Sirsha Asana. Those who are not able to perform Sirsha Asana can very well do this and derive the same benefits of Sirsha Asana. If Sirsha Asana is not done properly the practitioner may have some adverse effect on his health, whereas Sarvanga Asana can easily be done by anybody without any harmful effects. This Asana is particularly good for persons who are taking up Yoga after the age of 40.

Asana No. 4

MATSYA ASANA

(*The Fish Posture*)

Technique

- Sit in Padma Asana. **(Picture 63)**
- Gradually bend backwards and lie on the back.
- Do not raise the knees locked up in Padma Asana. Rest the elbows on the floor.
- Then bend the head backwards and make an arch form by bending the backbone.
- After bending the backbone in an arch, rest the head on the floor.
- For making a bigger arch exert more pull on the thighs and more twist on the neck and back. But do not strain to achieve.
- After making an arch of the body, stay in this position for ten to fifteen seconds. **(Picture 23)**
- An advanced way of doing this Asana is to bring the right hand below the body to the opposite side and catch the right big toe.
- Similarly the left hand should be brought below near the hip to catch the left big toe. **(Picture 24)**

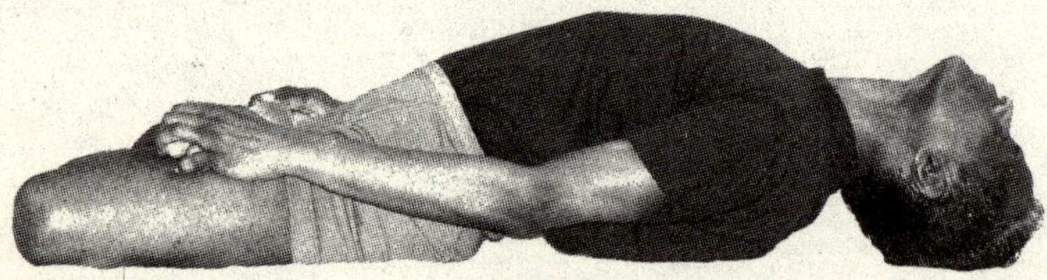

23
Matsya Asana

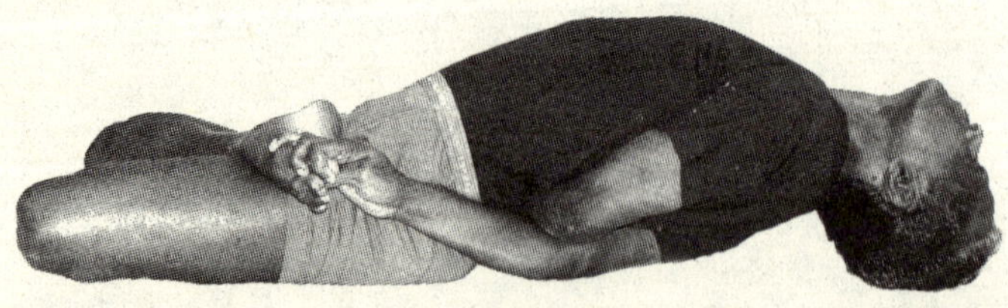

24
Matsya Asana
(Second Variation)

Synchronisation of Breath

Maintain normal breathing.

Benefits

- Activates the spine and all muscles of the back.
- Gives massage effect to facial tissues and face wrinkles disappear, thereby ensuring a youthful look.
- Removes stiffness of the neck and back and brings flexibility to the whole upper area of the body.
- As the chest is thrown open, deep breathing is possible. Helps to remove spasm from bronchial tubes and thereby relieves asthma.
- Backward pressure of the head causes a brisk flow of blood to all areas of the neck.
- An excellent Asana for colds and purulent tonsils.
- Thyroids and parathyroids receive lot of blood.
- Gives strength to the waist, back and neck.
- Tones up pituitary and pineal glands that are located in the brain.
- Eliminates constipation and massages abdominal organs.
- Good for women as it stimulates pelvic organs, especially genital ones and the ovaries in particular.
- Broadens the chest, corrects a hunchback and thereby ensures body symmetry.
- Good for wrestlers in preventing defeat by pin fall.
- Reduces fat from buttocks and stomach.
- Imparts lightness and activity to the body as a whole.
- Useful for abdominal illness.
- Helps diabetics by improving general metabolism.
- Relieves inflamed and bleeding piles.

Activates the Subconscious Mind

Since this Asana ensures varied benefits one should mentally repeat any statement suited to his needs.

Suitability

Suitable for all.

Precautions

None.

Asana No. 5

HAL ASANA

(The Plough Posture)

Technique

- Lie flat on the back full length.
- Place arms on both sides of the floor, palms facing the ground.
- Join both legs and lift them up slowly as you inhale. Do not bend your legs.
- Slowly raise the hips and lumbar region of the back.
- Lower the legs until the toes touch the floor beyond the head.
- Keep legs straight.
- Relax the body and remain in the final posture for a comfortable period of time. **(Picture 25)**

Another variation of this posture is to stretch both the hands behind the back. **(Posture 26)**

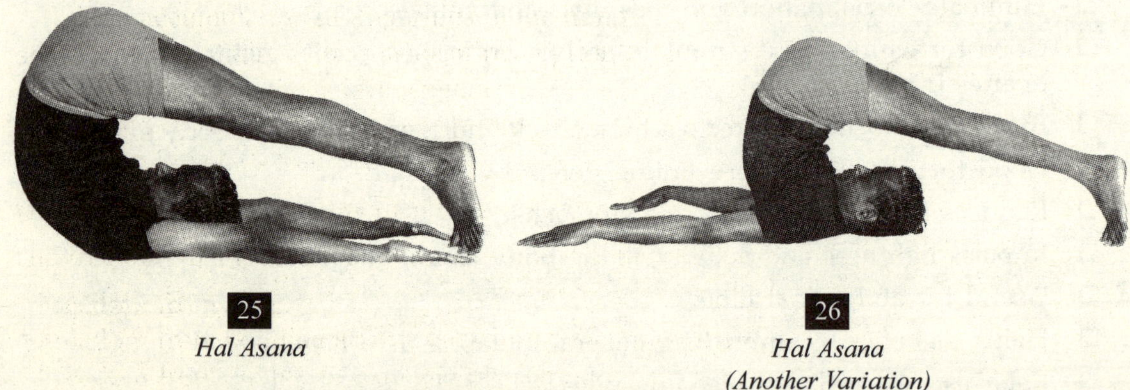

25 *Hal Asana*

26 *Hal Asana (Another Variation)*

Synchronisation of Breath

- Inhale when raising the legs.
- Exhale when lowering legs to the floor.
- Ensure normal breathing in the final posture.

Benefits

- ❑ According to Tantra Yoga, this Asana is one of the best to hone sexual powers. It invigorates and nourishes all sexual glands and thereby improves sexual potential to a considerable extent. It also corrects impotence, frigidity and lack of sexual powers.
- ❑ Activates functioning of abdominal organs, especially the kidneys and pancreas.

- Eliminates constipation, cures dyspepsia and improves digestion.
- Regulates activities of the thyroid and ensures agility and energy.
- The spine receives an extra supply of blood due to the forward bend and this relieves backache.
- Improves blood circulation in the brain, thereby contributing to intelligence, alertness and good memory.
- Cures certain types of diabetes as it helps to improve secretion of all glands in the abdomen.
- Corrects menstrual disorders in women.
- Prevents early ossification of vertebral bones.
- Cures enlargement of liver and spleen.
- Activates abdominal and rectal muscles as well as the thighs.
- Reduces fat from all parts of the body, especially the waist. Makes the body lighter and more active.
- Reduces muscular tension.
- Cures gastric and other stomach troubles.
- Eliminates piles.
- Reduces tendency towards high blood pressure.

Activate the Subconscious Mind

The benefits derived from this Asana are varied, so the practitioner may pick any benefit he would like to derive and concentrate on that particular aspect while performing this Asana. However, women suffering from frequent menstrual disorders may suggest to themselves that they are being cured of their menstrual problems after performing this Asana regularly. While doing this Asana, it is also good to suggest improvement in all sexual aspects.

Suitability

Suitable for all.

Precautions

Aged persons and those suffering from back pain and high blood pressure should not do this Asana.

Asana No. 6

CHAKRA ASANA

(*The Wheel Posture*)

Technique

- Lie on the back with feet well apart.
- Bend legs and arms and place palms on the floor a little behind the head, fingers pointing towards the feet. With some effort, raise the body above the ground and make an arch. **(Picture 27)**
- The entire body must rest on the feet and hands.

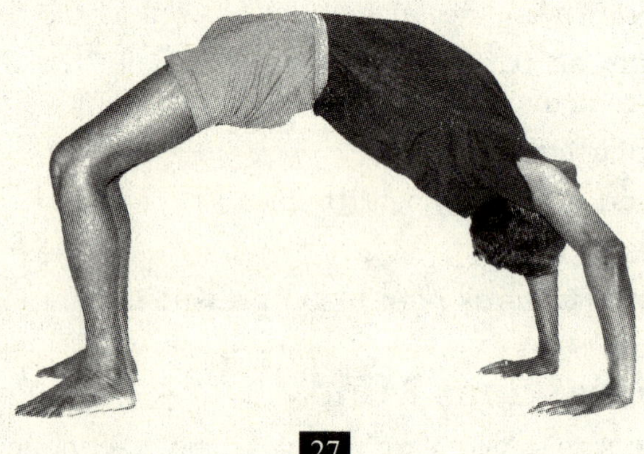

27

Chakra Asana

Synchronisation of Breath

Inhale while raising the body from the ground and making an arch. Retain breath in that position as long as possible. Exhale when resuming the normal position. Once mastery in performing this Asana is attained, one can stay in this posture for a longer duration with normal breathing.

Benefits

- ❑ Keeps the spine flexible even in old age.
- ❑ Beneficial for the entire nervous and glandular system.
- ❑ Develops muscles of back, neck, spine and shoulders.
- ❑ Activates the intestine.
- ❑ Keeps the practitioner alert and energetic.
- ❑ Sharpens eyesight.
- ❑ Improves texture and complexion of skin.
- ❑ Tones up the sex centre in the spine.

- Affords relief in constipation, flatulence and asthma.
- Tones up nerves serving the organs of sight, hearing, smell and taste.
- Controls gastric trouble.
- Energises a sluggish liver.
- Improves blood circulation to the brain and enhances intelligence and alertness.

Activate the Subconscious Mind

Those suffering from gastric trouble and sluggish liver may use autosuggestion to cure such ailments.

Suitability

Suitable for young boys and girls.

Precautions

None.

Asana No. 7

BHUJANGA ASANA

(*The Cobra Position*)

Special Note

This is one of the postures in Surya Namaskar **(Picture 7)**. However, it is presented separately because of its importance. This can be performed independently too.

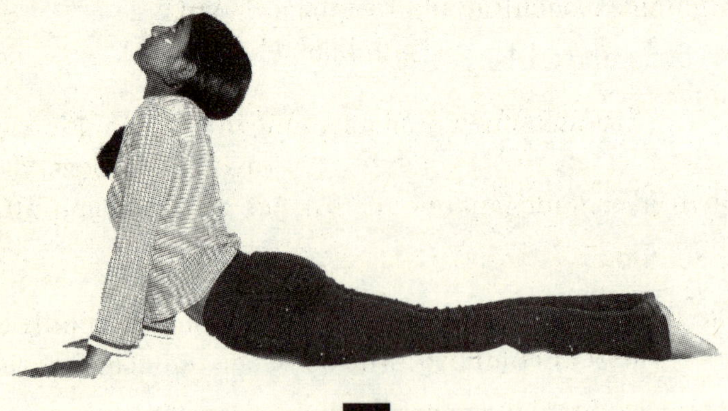

7

Bhujanga Asana

Technique

- Lie flat on the abdomen.
- Bring palms beneath the shoulder on both sides.
- Stretch legs straight to their full length, keeping them close together.
- Keep toes pointing outward.
- The head should be raised, giving a backward bend to the neck.
- The chest should be raised slowly, contracting the muscles of the back and the vertebral column (backbone) should be made to undergo an extension as much as possible.
- Keep the navel on the floor or close to the floor. The body above the navel area should be raised in an upward position.
- Now bring the arms into action and slowly bend the whole back as much as possible without straining until the arms are straight.
- Retain the posture for a while.
- Now lower the head gradually and return to the normal position.
- Repeat this process three to five times.

Synchronisation of Breath

Breathe in while bending backward, have inner retention while in the final posture and exhale while returning to the normal position.

Benefits

- Relieves pain in the back caused by overwork.
- The abdominal muscles are pulled and thereby strengthened.
- Increases inter-abdominal pressure.
- Raises body heat and destroys many ailments.
- Good for injured and slightly displaced spinal discs. Puts discs in their original position.
- The spinal region is toned.
- The chest is expanded.
- Reduces abdominal fat.
- Relieves constipation and flatulence and cures indigestion, dysentery, stomach ache and other abdominal problems.
- Helps overcome longstanding spinal pain even when caused by osteoarthritic changes in spine.
- Tones up muscles, tendons and ligaments, as well as nerves and blood vessels of the spinal region.
- Brings suppleness to the spine, which is the source of health, vitality and youthfulness.
- Aids in normal functioning of thyroid gland if there has been any departure from the normal.
- Tones up supra-renal medulla, which manufactures adrenalin, the hormone promoting energy.
- Helps cure female sexual disorders like leucorrhoea (white discharge), dysmenorrhoea (painful or difficult menstruation) and also tones up the ovaries and uterus.
- The thoracic cavity is widened and allows full expansion of the lungs, thereby increasing breathing power.
- During the final posture the gallbladder, spleen and pancreas are stimulated by the gentle and deep massage.
- Promotes beauty and increases feminine charm.
- Regular practise makes childbirth easy.
- Awakens Kundalini Shakti.
- Sexual performance of men and women is considerably improved as this Asana provides superb exercise to the spinal sex centre.

- Activates chest, shoulder, neck, face and head areas in an effective way, enhancing facial beauty.

Activate the Subconscious Mind

This Asana is particularly suited for toning up the spine and regular practise makes the spine supple and flexible. Since the suppleness of spine ensures radiant vitality and youthfulness one may concentrate on this aspect and use the following autosuggestion while performing the Asana:

"I am gaining radiant health and a youthful look."

Suitability

Suitable for all, but ensures greater benefits for ladies.

Asana No. 8

YOGA MUDRA ASANA

(*Yoga Seal Posture*)

Special Remarks

This Asana is highly extolled in Yogic literature for awakening the Kundalini Shakti. Remaining in this posture for a long time awakens the dormant Shakti.

Technique

Sit in Padma Asana or Sukha Asana. Hold the hands back and raise as much as possible **(Picture 28)**. While exhaling, slowly bend forward, bringing the forehead to the floor. Remain in this posture as long as you feel comfortable. Inhale and assume the original sitting posture. Repeat thrice.

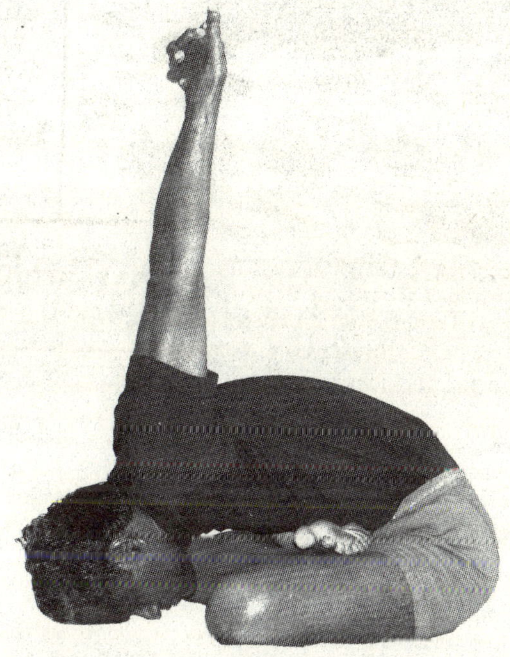

28

Yoga Mudra Asana

Synchronisation of Breath

While bending forward breathe out and have outer retention in the final posture. While raising the head up, breathe in.

Benefits

- Raising the hands up expands the chest and increases the range of shoulder movements.
- The pressure of the folded hands and bending forward stimulates the pancreas, liver and spleen.
- Ensures suppleness of the spine, increases digestive power, prevents pot belly, removes fat, eliminates constipation and improves blood circulation to the head.

Activate the Subconscious Mind

Focus the attention on one of the benefits of this Asana.

Suitability

Suitable for all, except those suffering from high blood pressure, who should avoid doing this.

Precautions

None.

Asana No. 9

BHADRA ASANA

(The Good Posture)

Technique

- ❑ Sit with both the legs fully stretched out.
- ❑ Fold both legs simultaneously and ensure the soles of the feet touch each other all along.
- ❑ Hold the feet with both hands and draw them nearer to the body trying to touch the genitals with the heels.
- ❑ Press both knees so that they touch the floor.
- ❑ Keep the upper part of the body and neck erect.
- ❑ Keep both hands on respective knees. **(Picture 29)**
- ❑ With the hands you may swing your legs up and down as many times as you feel comfortable. This is also called **Butterfly Posture**.
- ❑ In the same posture, bend forward and touch the ground with the forehead. This is the final posture. **(Picture 30)**

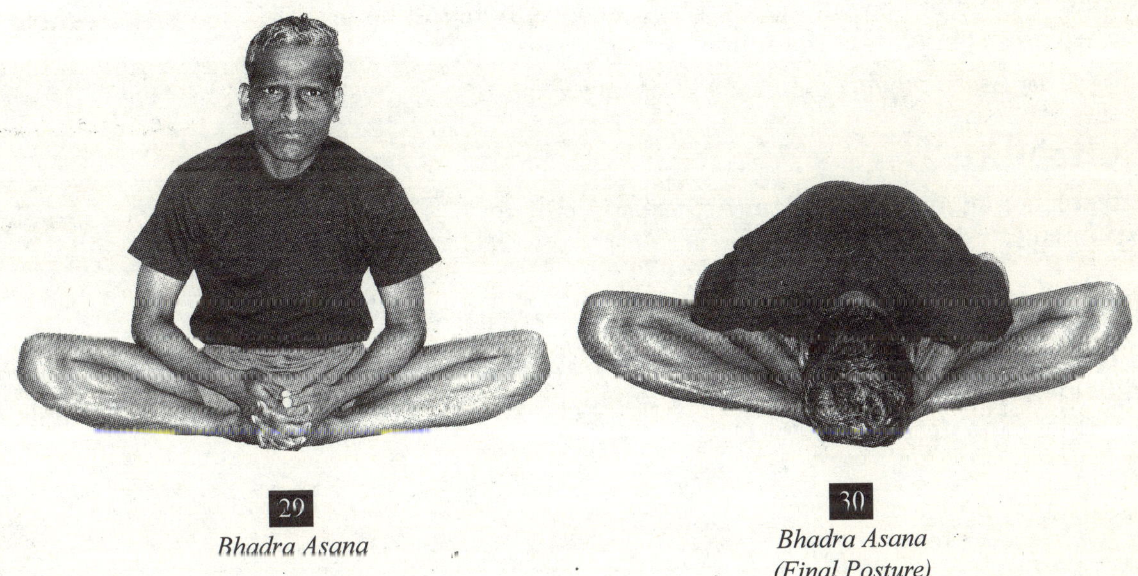

29
Bhadra Asana

30
Bhadra Asana (Final Posture)

Synchronisation of Breath

Maintain normal breath.

Benefits

- Makes legs and feet very flexible.

- Exercises both superficial and deep muscles of the inner side of thigh.
- Strengthens muscles and ligaments of uro-genital region.
- Prevents erotic dreams and involuntary discharge.
- Tones up nerves, muscles and circulatory system of the perineum and the genital organs of both men and women.
- Improves quality of seminal fluid.
- Improves sexual performance considerably.
- Eliminates premature ejaculation and maintains erection of penis in males during coitus for a considerable length of time.
- Strengthens the circulatory and neuromuscular system of the female uro-genital organs and improves chances of conception.

Activate the Subconscious Mind

Since this Asana considerably improves sexual performance in males, those who cannot effectively perform the sexual act may derive maximum benefit from this Asana by the following autosuggestion:

"My sexual performance is improving considerably through this Asana."

Those ladies who did not conceive even after a few years of marriage may do this Asana with great benefit and chances of conception will be bright if one practises this Asana consistently. Use the following suggestion:

"This Asana improves my chances of conception."

Suitability

Suitable for all, but an excellent Asana especially for a person seeking to improve sexual potential.

Precautions

While doing this Asana, both the knees should touch the ground. If this is not possible initially, the attempt should be made gradually by pressing both knees with the hands to achieve the desired result.

Asana No. 10

ARDHA MATSYENDRA ASANA

(Half Spinal Twist Posture)

Technique

- Sit with legs stretched in front.
- Bend the left leg and place under buttocks so that the upper end of the heel touches the upper end of the thigh. Place right hand behind the back.
- Hold toe of the right leg with left hand.
- The left hand should be straight and kept outside the right knee.
- Twist body towards right as much as possible.
- Remain in this posture for 10 to 15 seconds. **(Picture 31)**
- Change position of legs and hands alternately and continue the same procedure. **(Picture 32)**

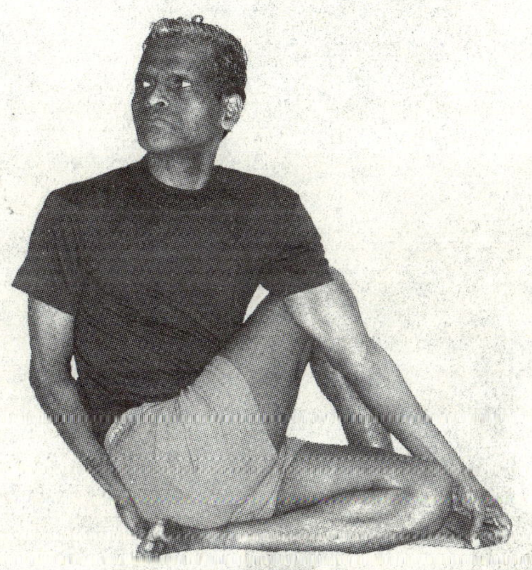

31

Ardha Matsyendra Asana

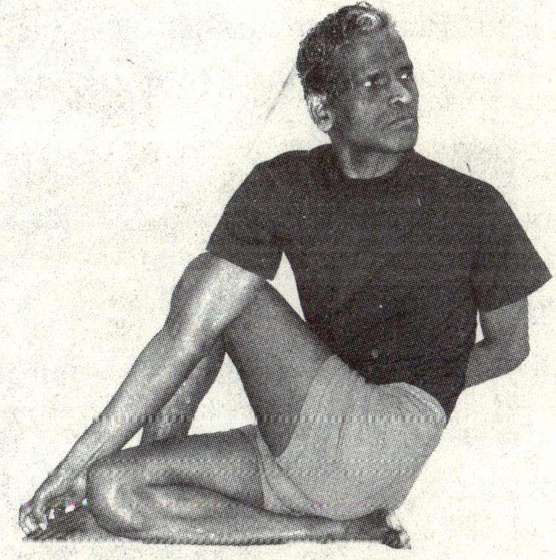

32

Ardha Matsyendra Asana
(Another Variation)

Synchronisation of Breath

- Exhale while twisting the entire body.
- Have normal breathing while maintaining final posture.
- Inhale while returning to the normal position.

Benefits

- Tones up pancreas, adrenal, thyroid and sex glands.
- Abdominal muscles are strengthened.
- Due to internal activation, disorders of kidneys, spleen, liver, stomach, intestine, bladder and pelvis are corrected.
- Provides maximum flexibility to the spine.
- Removes spinal pain and tones up spinal nerves.
- Compresses abdominal area, thereby eliminating constipation and dyspepsia and improving digestion.
- Protects against enlargement of prostrate and bladder.
- Good for persons with weak kidneys experiencing urinary troubles.
- Tones up sexual organs and greatly improves sexual performance of both men and women.
- Ensures beneficial results for diabetics.

Activate the Subconscious Mind

As it is a good posture for diabetes, diabetics may suggest as follows:

"I am getting relief from diabetes."

Suitability

Suitable for all but especially good for diabetics.

Precautions

Initially, it is difficult to hold the toe of the right leg with the left hand as described. However, this should be achieved gradually to derive maximum benefit.

Asana No. 11

PASCHIMOTHAN ASANA

(Back Stretching Posture)

Technique

- Lie flat on the back with arms parallel to the body and legs together.
- Inhale deeply and stiffen the body.
- Slowly raise the head and chest and assume a sitting posture, keeping the knees rigid and legs on the floor.
- Now exhale and bend further to hold the toe.
- Then slowly bend till the face rests on the knees. **(Picture 33)**
- Inhale and return to the sitting position and then be flat on your back with arms parallel to the body.

This Asana could be done in a dynamic manner and can be repeated three to five times.

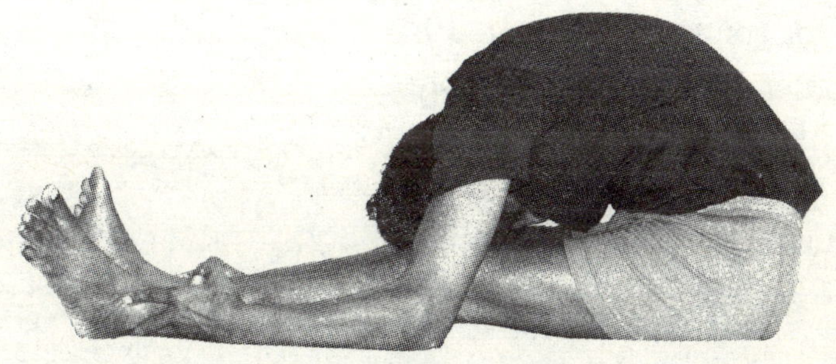

33

Paschimothan Asana

Synchronisation of Breath

As explained above.

Benefits

- Brings flexibility to the spine. According to Yoga, the rigidity of the spine is a symptom of old age. So flexibility ensures qualities of youthfulness.
- Corrects all disorders of the spine.
- Relieves backache and back problems.
- Abdominal muscles and organs are toned up.
- Cures all kinds of stomach trouble. This is one of the best postures to improve digestion. It is stated in the Vedas that a person can consume poison and do this

Asana. The poison will be digested. However, we advise readers NOT to risk trying this experiment.

- Good for those with low blood pressure.
- Removes excess fat from the stomach and hips.
- Tones up the lumber region of the spine.
- The solar plexus and nervous system of the spine are gently stimulated and freed from congestion.
- Renews vigour and vitality in sexual activity and removes disorders of the pancreas, liver, gallbladder, kidneys, intestines, spleen and seminal secretions.
- Prevents certain forms of ulcers.
- The waist is reduced, as adipose tissue is removed from the stomach and thighs, thereby improving physical personality.
- Especially good for ladies as it reduces excess fat and develops a graceful figure.
- Increases height if practised in adolescence.
- Alleviates muscular pains, especially in lumber and dorsal regions as well as the legs.
- Advocated for controlling repeated hiccups and asthmatic attacks.
- Improves general health considerably.

Activate the Subconscious Mind

Since there are innumerable benefits derived from this Asana it is better to choose one of the benefits according to one's need. Persons with weak digestive capacity may suggest to themselves that their digestive power is increasing.

Those desirous of developing a graceful figure may concentrate on this aspect. Persons suffering from stomach disorders and constipation may mentally repeat that they are greatly relieved from stomach trouble.

Suitability

It is suitable for all. However, people with weak digestive power may secure more beneficial results. It is good for ladies in attaining a graceful figure, and for the middle-aged to improve their sex lives.

Precautions

People with slipped discs and those suffering from sciatica, chronic arthritis and sacral infections should not perform this Asana.

Asana No. 12

MAYUR ASANA

(*Peacock Posture*)

Technique

- Lie down on the stomach.
- Raise the entire body from the ground keeping the elbows on the stomach.
- The entire body should be supported on the toes and palms. (Preparatory Posture – **Picture 34**)
- Now slowly lift both legs up.
- Initially, it is very difficult to raise both legs. In such cases, keep one leg on the ground and raise the other leg.
- Gradually try to raise both legs and balance the whole body on the elbows only.
- The body should be in a somewhat slanting position.
- The position of the head should be lower than the legs.
- Remain in this posture for 20 to 30 seconds. (Final Posture – **Picture 35**)

Those adept at Padma Asana can assume Padma Mayur Asana **(Picture 36)**.

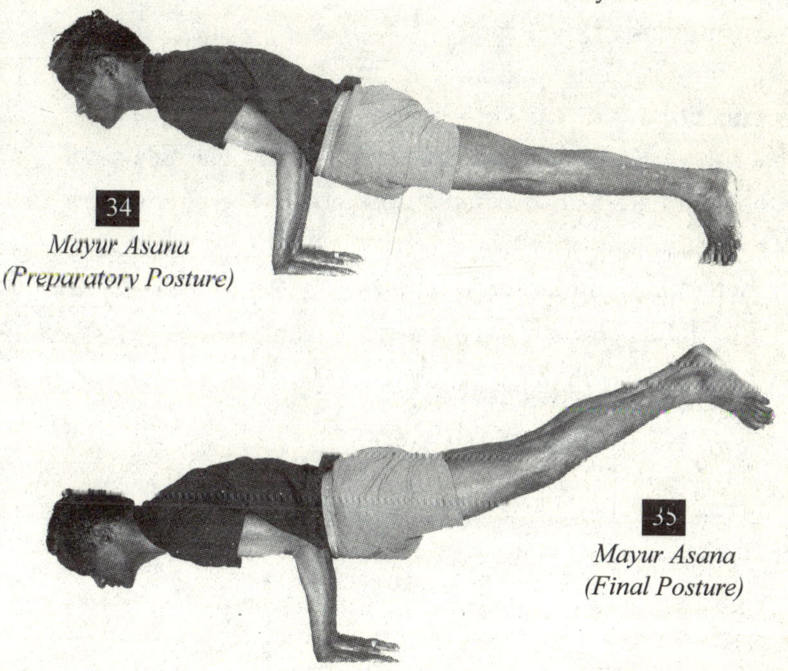

34 *Mayur Asana (Preparatory Posture)*

35 *Mayur Asana (Final Posture)*

Synchronisation of Breath

Inhale while raising legs upwards. Maintain normal breath in final posture.

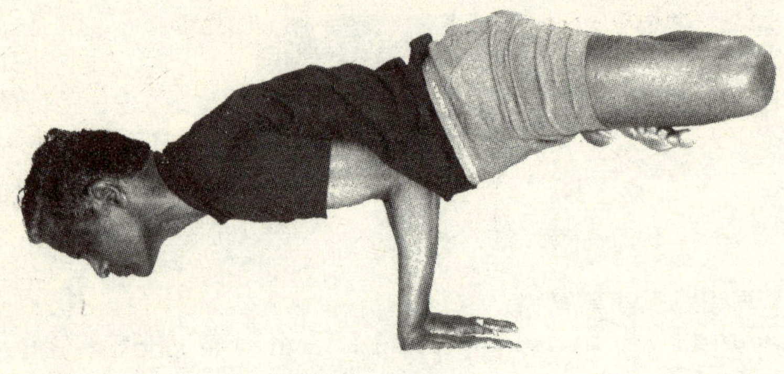

36

Padma Mayur Asana

Benefits

- The lungs and abdominal organs are toned up.
- Activates functioning of liver.
- Improves appetite.
- Destroys the effects of unwholesome food.
- Cures dyspepsia and chronic gastritis.
- Cures diabetes.
- Strengthens muscles of the arms.
- Cures every type of constipation.
- Improves functioning of the spleen.
- Prevents accumulation of toxins caused by faulty eating habits.
- Destroys poisonous effects created in the body.
- Increases breathing capacity.
- Helps remove skin complaints like boils.
- Awakens Kundalini Shakti.

Activate the Subconscious Mind

Concentrate on one of the benefits of this Asana.

Suitability

Suitable for all.

Precautions

Those suffering from high blood pressure, peptic ulcers and hernia should not perform this Asana.

Initially, it is better to keep a soft pillow below the head to avert hurting the nose.

Asana No. 13

SHAVA ASANA

(*Posture of Tranquillity*)

Technique

- Lie down on your back.
- Keep hands on the ground by the sides.
- The entire body should be kept relaxed and in a straight position.
- The eyes must be closed throughout this Asana.
- Now relax all muscles of the body.
- No part of the body should make the slightest movement. **(Refer to Picture 13)**
- No tension should remain in any part of the body.
- If someone were to raise the arm or leg they fall as if there is no life in them.
- For the time being, give up thinking about problems of daily life.
- Imagine you are sinking into the ground.
- Breathe normally and while exhaling let the mind feel that the body is going deeper down into the earth.
- One must be aware that one is relaxing and should not fall asleep.
- Consciously relax every part of the body and mentally direct the blood to a particular part of the body and after consistent practice one may feel that quite a good quantity of blood rushes to the specific body part where it has been directed. This area is then completely relaxed. This process of relaxation may be done from toes to face.
- Even in the face, one may practise relaxation of every part like the eyes, ears, and nose.
- When all the nerves are calmed down, one feels completely relaxed and refreshed.
- If relaxation is perfect and complete, one may feel the energy flows from the back of the head towards the heels.

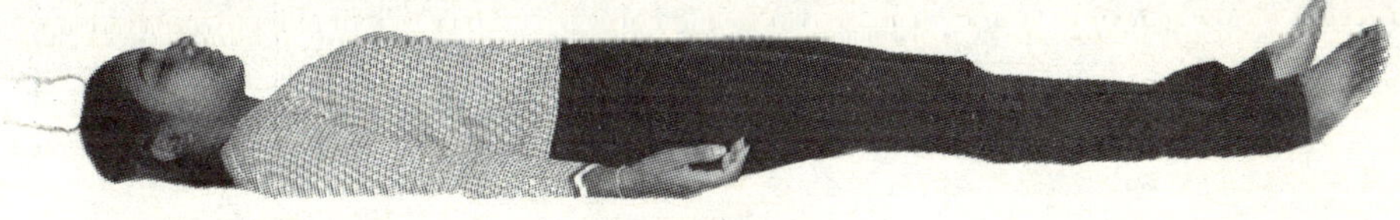

13

Shava Asana

This Asana may appear the easiest but is the most difficult to perform accurately. If a person trains himself to do this Asana correctly he derives immense benefit.

The best way for quick relaxation is to breathe out and pause. The time spent in **outer retention** is the point of relaxation. Breathe in, breathe out and pause – this is one cycle. If one wants total relaxation, one may repeat this cycle 20 to 25 times.

Synchronisation of Breath

Maintain normal breathing throughout this Asana. However, you should be fully conscious of your breathing process.

When the outer retention method is followed, then do as stated herewith.

Benefits

- Ensures complete relaxation and perfect ease. Removes fatigue in all situations.
- Induces calmness of mind.
- Best antidote for stresses of modern life. When the muscles, nerves and other organs are fully relaxed they gain strength and normal health is restored.
- Reduces blood pressure.
- Cures insomnia.
- Enables a practitioner to be satisfied with fewer hours of sleep.
- Turns the mind inwards and makes one introspective.
- Acts as a prophylactic against heart diseases in general. Eminent modern cardiologists worldwide prescribe this posture to speed up recovery of patients convalescing from heart diseases.
- If performed perfectly, the feeling of relaxation from this Asana is far superior to that experienced from tranquillisers and sedatives.

Activate the Subconscious Mind

Suggestion plays an important role here. Be very conscious of directing the suggestion to relax each and every part of the body. It is also beneficial to have a common suggestion while doing this Asana.

"I am relaxing completely and all my muscles and nerves are fully relaxed."

Suitability

Suitable for all, but particularly good for those leading a life of stress and strain.

Precautions

It is quite likely that one may be prone to fall asleep initially. This must be consciously avoided.

Concluding Remarks

The 13 Asanas (postures) presented above are known as **'classical Asanas'**. The practise of these will ensure profound benefits. I practise these Asanas regularly and consistently in the same order they are presented here. It takes about 30 minutes to perform them. The practise of these Asanas will bring sound health for the practitioner.

Youngsters should learn to practise all these Asanas. Adults may confine themselves only to the easy ones, depending upon ability and flexibility of body. **Surya Namaskar is a must for all.**

Part Three

Theory and Practise of Pranayama

PRANAYAMA THEORY

Introduction

The best way to **generate abundant energy and vitality** is through the practise of Pranayama.

In all my training programmes I ask participants: "Where is life located in our body?" I receive a variety of answers such as: "In the heart," "in the brain," "in the lungs" or "it pervades the whole body". Then I promise to demonstrate where life is located in my body by closing my nose and mouth, thereby stopping my breathing for a few seconds.

Then I have to remove my hand from the nose and inform them, "If life were located in my body, I would continue to live. The mere fact that I cannot hold my breath for a long time indicates that life is not in our body. We draw life from the atmosphere through the process of breathing. The atmosphere is filled with the life force called Prana. There is constant interaction between *Purusha* (human beings) and *Prakriti* (the atmosphere) through the process of breathing. The life force is freely available to all of us. Unfortunately, breathing is taken for granted. Many do not know the correct technique to draw more Prana from the atmosphere."

Concept of Prana

'Prana' refers to the vital force pervading the entire universe and representing the principle of cosmic energy. It exists in all forms from the highest to the lowest, both in animate and inanimate objects. Everything in this world owes its existence to the presence of Prana. It is responsible for the growth process in this world. It is the same Prana that manifests in the form of electricity, gravity, magnetism etc. It is manifested as the actions of the human body, as the nerve currents and also as a thinking force. From thought down to the lowest force, everything is nothing but the manifestation of Prana.

Definition of Pranayama

Ancient *rishis* and Yogis in India innovated a variety of techniques to draw more Prana from the atmosphere and also to preserve excess Prana in the solar plexus. In normal breathing, our intake of Prana is very little. The techniques innovated in this regard are called *Pranayama.*

Yama denotes *to control. Prana* refers to the life force. Pranayama is the control of bio-energy (life force) through the respiratory system.

Pranayama denotes a pause in the movement of breath, referring to the process of control of the life force through the act of breathing.

It may be defined as a systematic approach designed to bring about perfect control over the flow of Prana throughout the body by the application of certain methods and techniques achieved through the regulation of physical breathing.

Pranayama Vs Deep Breathing

The main objective of any deep breathing exercise is the absorption of oxygen into the body to the maximum extent. It is practised via vigorous exercise of one type or another and the absorption of oxygen is compensated by the energy expended in the exercise. Pranayama also involves breathing exercises. However, it is undertaken in a relaxed posture, with a serene attitude, without any jerky movements and, therefore, the intake of oxygen in the body outbalances the energy spent.

By and large, people do not breathe properly. Therefore, a large quantity of air remains in the lower lobes of the lungs. This residual air is not expelled through ordinary deep breathing exercise. One of the essential features of Pranayama is the introduction of inner and outer retentions (i.e., Anthara and Bhahkya Kumbakha). During inner retention, the concentration of carbon dioxide in the air cells of the lungs is diluted and with forced expelling followed by retention a large quantity of carbon dioxide is removed. Again, deep inhalation followed by expelling would facilitate the lungs being filled with fresh air and, thereby, the quantum of air at the residue level is considerably changed.

During Pranayama, the production of carbon dioxide is very negligible, as it does not involve physical exertion and mental strain, which generally result in tiredness. In the absence of such tiredness, Pranayama can be prolonged to a considerable extent, further facilitating complete removal of carbon dioxide from the air cells of the lungs. This is not possible with ordinary deep breathing exercises.

Pranayama brings about inner, organic and natural harmony. This is possible through alternate breathing. According to Yoga, there are two sets of bio nervous (Prana, Apana Vayus) influences that cause and control the act of respiration. They are called Surya (positive solar influence created by breathing through the right nostril) and Chandra (negative lunar influence caused by breathing through the left nostril). When coordination is ensured between these two vital biodynamic currents, a wholesome balance is achieved in the human body, which is highly responsible for sound health. With ordinary deep breathing exercises, this coordination is not possible, as it does not involve alternate breathing.

Ordinary deep breathing is intended to develop a big chest. This is not very useful for maintaining good health. The health and dynamism of the body depends mainly upon the quantity and quality of blood circulating throughout the system. In Pranayama, a large volume of blood is arterialised with each respiration. This facilitates the intake of air reaching each and every cell in the body. Arterialisation is not possible unless deep breathing is followed with increased pulmonary circulation. This is possible only in Pranayama.

Prana and Oxygen

Prana represents energy, whereas oxygen is a substance. In a scientific laboratory, Prana cannot be isolated and identified, whereas oxygen can be separated from other substances. The atmospheric air contains oxygen charged with Prana, which is the vital force that sustains human life. The life force (Prana) in the living being is called *Purusha*, while that in the universe is known as *Prakriti*. There is constant interaction between *Purusha* and *Prakriti* through the process of breathing. The life force reaches every cell of the human body through the oxygen we breathe in with air – that is, from *Prakriti*. The moment the interaction between these two is severed (when breathing ceases), the living being embraces death. Oxygen is not the life force. It is only a vehicle to carry Prana, just as a wire transmits electric power.

Therefore, we may logically conclude that if more oxygen is absorbed into our body through Pranayama, more Prana would automatically enter our body. However, if only oxygen were necessary to keep all physiological functions running, a dead man would come to life if given oxygen in the required quantity.

Different Methods of Respiration

Indian Yogis have classified respiration into (a) high breathing, (b) mid breathing, (c) low breathing, and (d) yogic complete breathing.

High breathing is known as **clavicular breathing** or **collarbone breathing**. In this form of respiration, the ribs, collarbone and shoulder are raised and the abdomen is drawn in. The upper part of the chest and lungs is used and as a result only a minimum amount of air enters the lower part of the lungs. This type of breathing may be practised by placing one hand on the upper chest just below the collarbone and breathing deeply in and out while directing the consciousness to breathe and fill the upper part of the lungs.

Mid breathing is called **rib breathing** or **inter-costal breathing**. In mid breathing, the diaphragm is pushed upwards and the abdomen drawn in. The ribs are raised to some extent and the chest is partially expanded. Here, the flow of air and Prana gets into the mid chest and heart area. Women are good mid breathers and, therefore, less prone to heart diseases than men. Mid breathing can be consciously developed by placing one hand on the chest between the breast and breathing deeply in and out.

Low breathing is called **abdominal breathing**, deep breathing or **diaphragmatic breathing**. This is the natural form of breathing but ladies are poor abdominal breathers. Here, the flow of air enters the area below the navel. In order to practise low breathing, place your hand on the diaphragm and breathe deeply in and out and consciously make an effort to pass air into the lowest part of the lungs.

In the above methods, only a part of the lungs is filled with air. Therefore, it is necessary to develop a habit of breathing in which we can fill our entire lungs and, thereby, the maximum quantity of oxygen is absorbed and, also, the maximum amount of Prana is stored in the nervous system. This is accomplished by **Yogic complete breathing**. Such breathing covers all good aspects of high breathing, mid breathing and low breathing. An important aspect of this method is that all respiratory muscles are fully called into play. In other types of respiration only a portion of the muscles are used.

Yogic complete breathing may be practised by placing one hand on the diaphragm and the second hand on the mid chest. The lower hand may be raised to the high chest area after the lower lobes are filled. During this process, the hands are placed in a way that facilitates consciousness to direct the flow of air to first enter the lower lobes of the lungs, then the middle and finally the high-chest area of the lungs. While breathing out, the air should come out first from the abdomen, then from the mid and high chest, respectively.

Yogic complete breathing is the foundation on which the entire edifice of the science of Pranayama has been constructed. Therefore, the Pranayama student should first thoroughly acquaint himself with it before wishing to obtain fruitful results from the other forms of Pranayama mentioned in this book.

Benefits of Pranayama

Pranayama begins with regulation of breath and ends in establishing full and **perfect control** over life-currents or the **inner vital force** (i.e. Prana).

Through Pranayama we can consciously regulate the **uniformity of our breath** and establish a **balance** between **positive and negative currents**. The inner life force is like a positive current of electricity and the outer life force is like a negative current. **Exhalation** is the **positive state** during which the energy absorbed is **distributed** to all parts of the body and with **inhalation** we are in a **negative, receptive state**.

The main aim of all Pranayama exercises is to consciously **direct the flow** of Prana to **all parts of the body uniformly** to revitalise all internal organs and, in course of time, reach a state of development enabling us to produce currents or life force consciously with a simple command to the mind.

Prana is absorbed from the atmosphere through the process of breathing. By regular practise of Pranayama it is possible to **absorb more Prana than that possible** via ordinary breathing. The **excess** Prana is **stored** in the brain and nerve centres, just as a battery stores electricity. A person who has stored a large supply of Prana will radiate strength and vitality all around.

When Prana is controlled through Pranayama the **mind** is automatically **controlled**. Similarly, when the mind is controlled through concentration and meditation, Prana is also controlled. There is an intimate **connection** between **mind, Prana and semen**. If the seminal energy is controlled by continence, the mind and Prana are spontaneously controlled. The **Nadis** (subtle channels of nerve passage via which Prana passes through the whole body) are **purified** by the practice of Pranayama. When the Nadis are purified, the body mechanism undergoes a thorough change. The eyes sparkle with lustre, the voice becomes sweet and melodious, the body radiates charm and poise. The digestive capacity is increased and perfect health is ensured.

The mind plays a predominant role in Pranayama. It should not be done mechanically. To derive maximum benefit, it is necessary to **consciously absorb** everything that takes place via the phenomenon of breathing. Therefore, it is essential to **establish rhythm in breathing**. After the rhythm is fully established, the practitioner should imagine that with each inhalation he is drawing in an increased supply of Prana from the universal supply, which will be taken up by the nervous system and stored in the solar plexus and with each exhalation Prana is distributed to all parts of the body.

Pranayama keeps the flow of Pranic currents in perfect working condition at the **proper voltages** required by different parts of the body. Just as electricity can be used for different purposes, Pranic currents also perform a variety of functions in different parts of the body most efficiently when the body is in perfect condition. Any **disturbance** in the proper flow of this **Pranic current** results in **disease** of one kind or another depending upon the nature of such disturbance. A regular practitioner of Pranayama, therefore, would **never suffer from any disease** throughout his life. He will always be energetic and enthusiastic. There is no need for him to drink or smoke to stimulate himself. He gets **sound sleep** as soon as he retires to bed. Even four to five hours of refreshing sleep are sufficient to provide enough rest to his body and mind.

It has been scientifically proved that practise of Pranayama **cures many diseases**. The deficiency of red corpuscles in the blood can be corrected and an abnormal increase in **eosinopholis** can be **reduced**. Even after a few months of practise, **patches in the lungs disappear**, a sluggish liver and bowel can be reactivated, the vitality index rises and hormonal as well as glandular imbalances rectified.

PRELIMINARY INSTRUCTIONS

Posture

Pranayama is best done in a meditative posture, preferably Padmasana (Picture 63) or Vajra Asana (Picture 40). Padmasana being difficult for beginners, it is better to practise Pranayama in Vajra Asana.

Time

An empty stomach is mandatory. Therefore, the best time for practise is before breakfast. If practised in the evening, keep a gap of at least five hours after consuming solid food. Before sunrise or after sunset is the ideal time.

Place

The ideal place for Pranayama is a secluded spot on the banks of a river or on the beach. The room where Pranayama is practised should be well ventilated but free from any sudden gust of wind and devoid of foul smell, smoke and dust.

Sequence

Any student of Yoga should necessarily practise meditation. This may be done very early in the morning after waking up and finishing the morning ablutions. Then, after a gap of half an hour or an hour, the Asanas may be practised. Immediately after completing the Asanas, Pranayama may be done. This sequence is meant for those who devote much time for meditation.

If a person is hard-pressed for time and can devote only 10 to 15 minutes for meditation, he may follow the sequence of Asanas, Pranayama and meditation. During Pranayama and meditation, the nerves are soothed. Hence, Asanas should not be attempted immediately after Pranayama and meditation.

Actual Practise

Pranayama should be done in such a way that rhythm is established. By breathing very slowly and more deeply one can easily establish a new rhythm automatically. Maintaining this rhythm throughout is a prerequisite. When inner retention (holding the breath after breathing in) is maintained for a longer duration than it can be comfortably held, the practitioner may have to hurriedly exhale and, thereby, the rhythm may be disturbed. The loss of rhythm would defeat the very purpose of Pranayama.

During retention the muscles of the face should not be twisted. This is an indication that one is going beyond his capacity to retain breath.

For measuring the time of inhalation and exhalation one may mentally count numbers. The ticking sound of an alarm clock would also help the practitioner keep perfect time. If a person wants to be very accurate, he may use a metronome. Observing the time is necessary only in the beginning. After a year or so, there is no need to observe the time, as the whole process will become automatic through force of habit.

Pranayama should be practised for at least 15 minutes daily without missing a single day. Only then will the benefits be derived fully. The practice may be stopped only during serious illness. In case a practitioner falls sick, he should not attribute his illness to the practise of Pranayama. Pranayama will never bring ill health but only foster good health and vitality.

A person should not experience tiredness during Pranayama. If he does so, it indicates some wrong practice. In this case, one should seek the help of an expert. There should always be a feeling of joy and exhilaration, not tiredness. During Pranayama the eyes are closed to facilitate concentration.

Secretions of saliva in the mouth should be swallowed before exhaling a breath and not during retention.

Cultivating the habit of performing a few simple Asanas and Pranayama daily after getting up from bed will drive away drowsiness in a person and enable him to start the day enthusiastically.

It is necessary to practise Shava Asana after the completion of one round of each item of Pranayama. This refreshes one's body and mind.

Some Precautions

- ❑ The advanced stage in the practise of Pranayama envisages gradual introduction of certain Bandhas (interlocking techniques), Mudras (digital and facial postures). These should be practised only under the guidance of a qualified instructor.
- ❑ Children below the age of 12 should not attempt advanced Pranayama. However, they may be encouraged to breathe in and out slowly and rhythmically.
- ❑ When retention of breath is introduced it may cause constipation. This is just a temporary phenomenon. Those suffering from eye and ear trouble should not attempt retention of breath.
- ❑ People addicted to smoking or drinking should not attempt advanced Pranayama. However, they may start with mild practices and may later give up such habits voluntarily.
- ❑ The rate of respiration is quicker in women than in men. Hence, women should consciously practise Pranayama in a slow, rhythmic manner.

Bandhas

Bandha literally means a *lock*. In Yoga, Bandhas are one type of postures in which certain organs or parts of the body are contracted and controlled in order to influence the vascular, nervous and glandular systems. One of the aims of Pranayama is to direct the flow of Prana to various parts of the body. When Bandhas are performed in conjunction with Pranayama, the flow of Prana is properly controlled and directed to specific areas without much dissipation. Bandhas are generally used in advanced Pranayama practice.

There are three main Bandhas that are important in Pranayama. They are:

1. Jalandhara Bandha
2. Uddiyana Bandha
3. Moola Bandha

1. Jalandhara Bandha (Chin Lock)

- This Bandha is generally performed along with Pranayama. Hence, this may be done in one of the meditative postures.
- Inhale deeply and retain the breath inside.
- Bend the head forward, contract the throat, stretch the neck and press the chin tightly against the chest, particularly the sternum. **(Picture 37)**
- The position may be held as long as the breath is retained inside.
- This can be practised when the breath is retained outside also.

When the throat is contracted, the two vocal cords situated in the larynx are also contracted.

This Bandha regulates the flow of blood and Prana to the heart, the glands in the neck and head together with the brain.

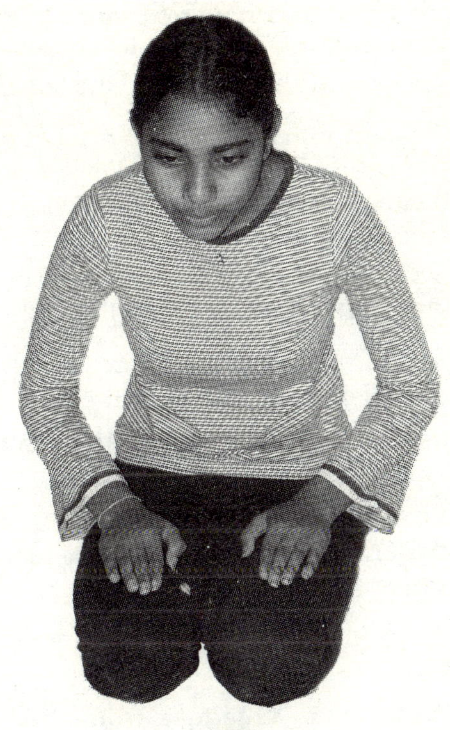

37

Jalandhara Bandha

When the breath is retained without this Bandha, the pressure will be felt immediately on the heart and the practitioner may feel dizzy.

The thyroid and parathyroid glands are massaged and their functioning improves. These glands play a vital role to improve the human organism, growth and sexual functions.

2. Uddiyana Bandha (Abdominal Retraction Lock)

- Assume a standing position keeping the legs apart. Bend and hold your right thigh with the right hand and the left thigh with the left hand.
- Exhale deeply and hold.
- Bend the head forward and do the Jalandhara Bandha.
- Next, pull the abdominal muscles inward as far as possible. (See **Picture 55**)
- This lock should be maintained as long as the breath is held.
- Slowly release the abdominal muscles, raise the head and take a slow, deep breath.

This Bandha cures all abdominal and stomach problems. It relieves constipation and indigestion.

All abdominal organs are toned and rendered more efficient. Some internal organs like the liver, pancreas, kidneys, spleen etc., are massaged and their functioning stimulated. Lethargic tendencies are driven away and an overactive person becomes tranquil.

This Bandha should not be performed after inhalation and inner retention.

Persons suffering from heart troubles and peptic ulcers should not do this Bandha. It is also prohibited for pregnant women.

3. Moola Bandha (Anal Contraction Lock)

- Assume the position of Vajra Asana.
- After deep inhalation, retain the breath inside.
- Now contract the muscles in the perineum and draw them upwards.

The correct performance of this Bandha increases sexual retentive power of the practitioner. It generates vitality and helps to awaken the Kundalini Shakti. The sphincter muscles of the anus are strengthened and intestinal peristalsis is stimulated. Constipation and piles are cured.

Practise of Pranayama

There are over a hundred Pranayama techniques, from which I have carefully selected only five, and practise them regularly everyday. I may skip breakfast but not the practise of Pranayama. My energy levels are very high on account of this. Therefore, I give below only those Pranayama techniques that I practise daily without fail. I earnestly urge readers to practise these techniques for maximum benefits in terms of tremendous energy, high enthusiasm and sound health.

These select five Pranayama techniques are:

1. Mukha Bastrika Pranayama (Yogic Cleansing Breath)

Technique

- Sit in Vajra Asana (**Picture 40**). Keep the palms on the respective thighs.
- Inhale fully through both nostrils.
- Next, forcibly exhale in a rapid succession of expulsions through your mouth by forming the Kaki Mudra (make a narrow tube with your lips). **(Picture 38)**
- As you exhale, bend forward and touch the ground with your forehead. If it is not possible for you to touch the ground, bend as far as possible. **(Picture 39)**
- Maintain the posture for a few seconds with outer retention. When you feel like breathing, lift your head up.
- Continue this process three to five times.

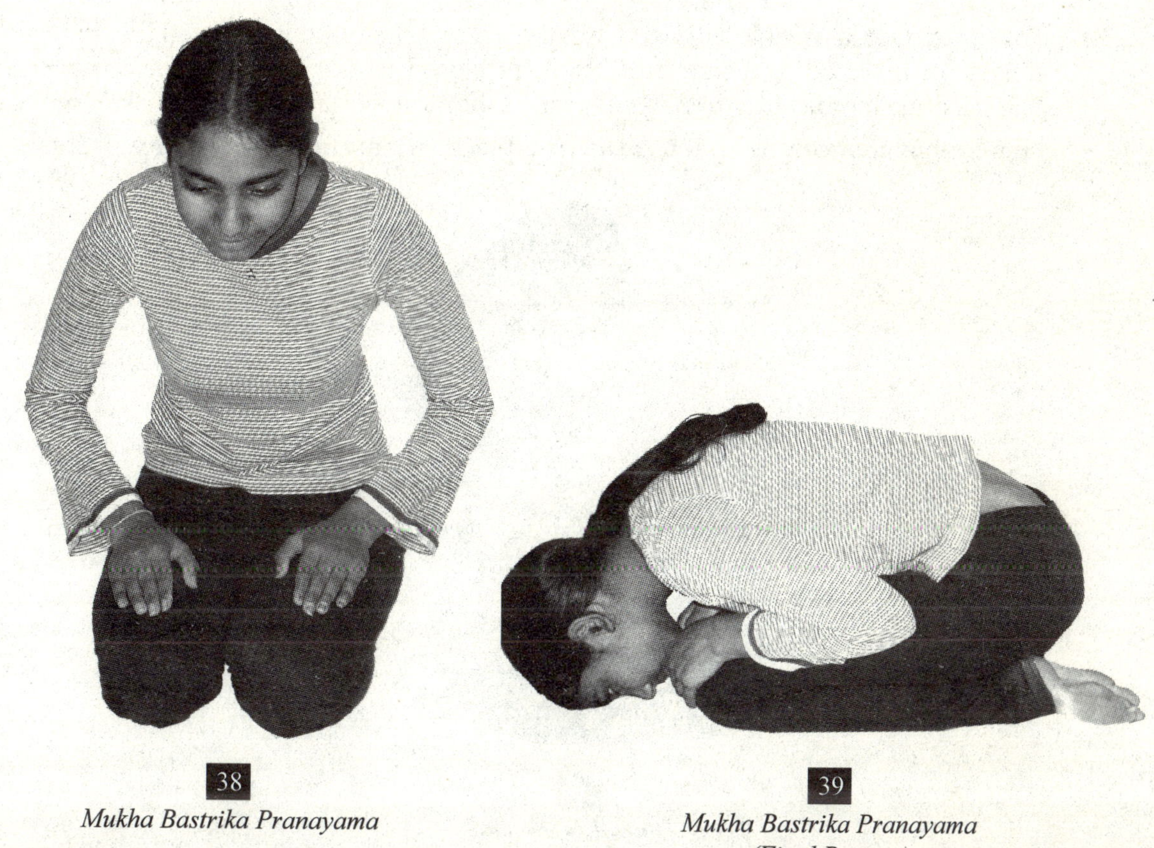

38

Mukha Bastrika Pranayama

39

Mukha Bastrika Pranayama
(Final Posture)

Benefits

- ❑ Very useful in ventilating and cleansing the lungs.
- ❑ Stimulates the cells and generally tones up the respiratory organs.

2. UJJAYI PRANAYAMA (Success Pranayama)

Technique

- Sit in Vajra Asana.
- Inhale through both nostrils by gently contracting the neck, the chin slightly touching the chest collarbone. The air will not have free flow, being obstructed in the pharyngeal area. There will be a sibilant sound when the air is passed through the back wall of the mouth. Though you breathe through both nostrils, it appears as if the nostrils are not used and they remain inactive in the entire process of this Pranayama. You have the sensation of breathing through the throat. **(Picture 40)**

- This Pranayama is characterised by the resonant sound produced by partial closure of the glottis, which must be kept closed throughout the performance. The frictional sound due to partial closure should be of a low but uniform pitch.
- This Pranayama can be practised in any place, at any time and in any posture.

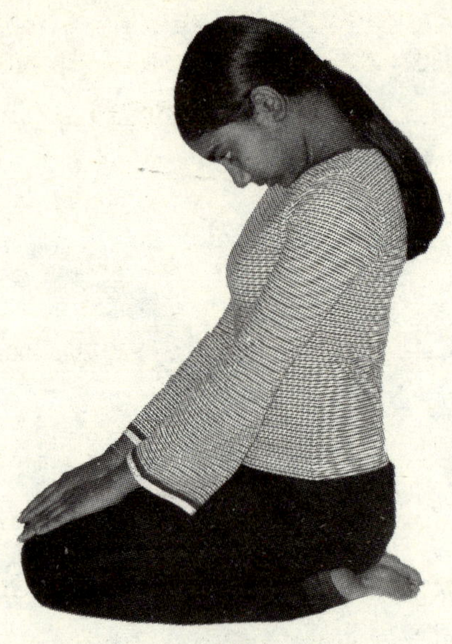

40

Ujjayi Pranayama

Benefits

- This Pranayama enables one to have a higher intake of Prana into the system. Due to partial closure of the glottis, the inhaled air will have friction, which generates energy. This is one of the best Pranayama techniques to generate more energy in a short time. I do this Pranayama very frequently everyday whenever I find time.
- Removes tiredness and fatigue. The more you practise, the greater the possibility of more energy.
- Relieves coughing, aerates the lungs, removes phlegm, soothes the nerves and tones up the entire nervous system.
- Highly beneficial for those with high blood pressure. They can do it in reclining position.

On many occasions I have experienced that phlegm is being removed from my chest. This Pranayama can be practised while travelling.

3. NADI SHODHANA PRANAYAMA (Alternate Breath Pranayama)

Technique

- Sit in Vajra Asana with the left arm on the left thigh. The thumb and ring finger of the right hand should gently touch each side of the nose, with the index and middle fingers on the forehead. **(Picture 41)**
- Close the right nostril with the thumb and inhale through the left nostril for a count of three. After inhalation close both nostrils and hold the breath with Jalandhara and Moola Bandhas for a count of six. Then release the Bandhas and exhale through the right nostril for a count of six. Then close both nostrils and have outer retention for a count of three. Now inhale through the right nostril for a count of three. Close both nostrils and have inner retention with Jalandhara and Moola Bandhas for a count of six. Then exhale through left nostril for a count of six and have outer retention for three counts. It completes one round of this Pranayama.
- Have three rounds initially and increase the number according to need and time available.

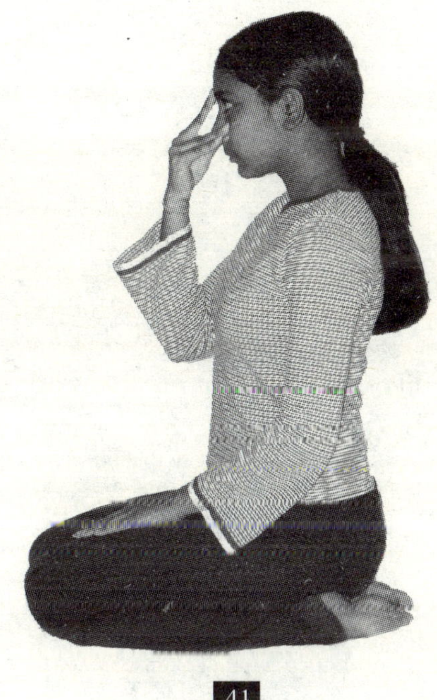

41

Nadi Shodhana Pranayama

Benefits

- ❑ Brings calmness and tranquillity and purifies the nerves. The bloodstream is purified of toxins and the blood receives a larger supply of oxygen than in normal breathing.

- Due to alternate breathing the flow of Prana in the Ida and Pingala Nadis is equalised. Right nostril breath stimulates the left hemisphere of the brain and left nostril breath activates the right hemisphere. This is one of the best Pranayama techniques that makes optimum use of both brain hemispheres. Most geniuses use both hemispheres of the brain.

4. KAPALABHATI PRANAYAMA (Brain Stimulating Pranayama)

Technique

- Sit in Vajra Asana. Close fists of both hands with the thumb inside and place them on the thighs touching each other. This is Maha Mudra. **(Picture 42)**
- Inhale in a mild, slow, long manner and exhale quickly and forcibly by contracting abdominal muscles with a backward push for as many times as possible. Inhalation and exhalation occur simultaneously. Inhalation is mild and silent and exhalation is forceful and vehement. There is no retention in this Pranayama.

Beginners can do it 20 to 30 times. This should be increased gradually. I do it everyday for 500 times at a stretch without break.

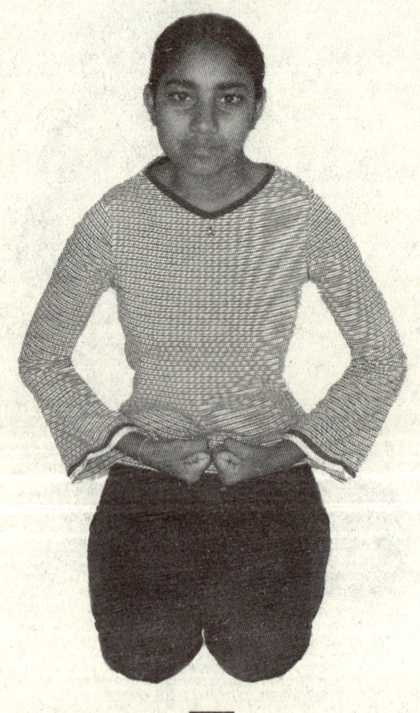

42

Kapalabhati Pranayama

Benefits

- Cleanses respiratory system and nasal passages.

- ❑ Asthma is relieved. Carbon dioxide is eliminated. Aids proper heart functioning.
- ❑ Every single cell in the brain is stimulated to an extraordinary level. One of the best techniques to improve intelligence and creativity.

5. BANDHATREYA PRANAYAMA (Preserve Excess Prana)

Technique

- Sit in Vajra Asana. Keep the eyes closed and the whole body relaxed.
- Breathe in deeply and softly as in Ujjayi Pranayama. Feel that you are breathing through the throat only.
- Hold the breath and do Jalandhara and Moola Bandhas.
- When Moola Bandha is performed, Uddhiyana Bandha takes place automatically.
- Stay in this position for as long as you can comfortably hold the breath inside with the Bandhas. (**Posture 43)**
- When you feel like breathing out take your chin up and exhale, releasing the Bandhas. This is one round. You may do 10 to 15 rounds.

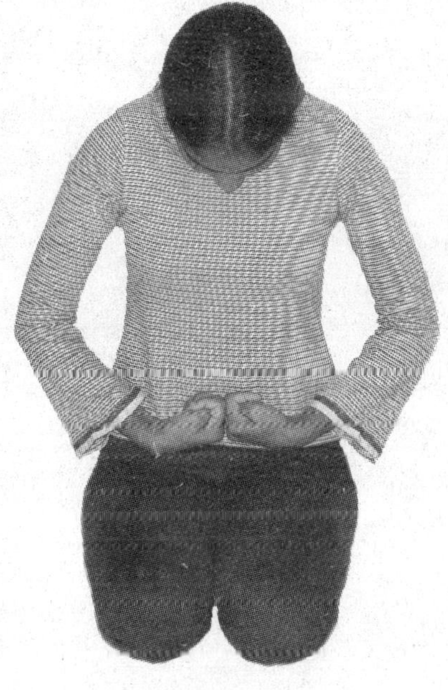

43

Bandhatreya Pranayama

Benefits

- ❑ Ensures strength and vitality.
- ❑ Preserves excess Prana in solar plexus, enabling the excess Prana to be utilised in times of need.

- Sexual glands are revitalised.
- Constant practise enables one to lead a healthy life.

After completing all the Pranayama techniques, lie on the ground and relax.

Relaxation may be done in the following manner: Breathe in and out slowly and then pause. This is outer retention called Bhakya Kumbakha. After breathing out, do not breathe in immediately. This is the point of relaxation. Be in this posture as long as you feel comfortable. Then breathe in. Do ten rounds of this relaxation exercise.

Part Four

Practices of Shat Karma

Shat Karma consists of six purificatory processes developed by ancient Hatha Yogis for the purpose of eliminating poisonous substances accumulated in various parts of the human body.

The body constantly expels waste matter in the form of perspiration, urine, excretion and breath through various mechanisms. If this waste matter is not properly and completely thrown out in the regular processes the body would be loaded with disease-carrying poisons. So, in order to maintain perfect health, it is necessary to purge all impurities from the body. This is achieved by the practise of Shat Karma, given below:

(1) Neti
- (a) Jala Neti
- (b) Sutra Neti

(2) Dhauti
- (a) Kunjala or Gajakarni
- (b) Vastra Dhauti
- (c) Varisara Dhauti or Shankha Prakshalana

(3) Basti

(4) Nauli

(5) Kapalabhati

(6) Trataka

(1) NETI

(a) Jala Neti

The main purpose of Jala Neti is to remove all dirt and bacteria-filled mucus from the nasal passages with lukewarm water.

This may be done as follows:

- Take a small half-litre capacity jug with a spout or nozzle. The size of the spout should be enough to enable inserting it into one's nostrils with ease. Fill the jug with pure lukewarm water and add one teaspoon of salt per half litre.
- Insert the spout in one of the nostrils, say, right nostril, and slightly tilt the head in the opposite direction so that the water comes out of the other (left) nostril. **(Picture 44)**

- During this process, breathe only through the mouth. If there is no blockage in the nostrils the water will flow easily. Otherwise, it will take some time to pass through the other nostril. In case the water does not come out at all from the other nostril, you should perform Sutra Neti, which will be explained later. You should also ascertain that the water passes only through the other nostril and should not enter the mouth. If it does, then the position of the head should be adjusted accordingly.
- After completing the exercise, stand erect and bend forward at an angle of 90 degrees and blow the left nostril with vigour as in Kapalabhati Pranayama so that the residue water in the nasal passage comes out from the right nostril.
- Repeat the process by inserting the spout in the left nostril and remove the water from the right nostril. Also do Kapalabhati Pranayama to remove residue water from the right nostril.
- When the process of passing water through both nostrils is complete, stand erect and do Kapalabhati Pranayama by breathing in and out vigorously through both nostrils about 25 to 30 times in succession, laying more emphasis on exhalation so that all the water from the nasal passage comes out and the nose is fully dry.

Next, perform **Shashanga Asana** as follows: **(Picture 45)**

- Sit in Vajra Asana. Bend the head forward and touch the floor with your forehead. Interlock hands and keep them on the back. Be in this posture for about two to three minutes. This Asana will remove any water droplets not removed by Kapalabhati Pranayama.

Those who attempt Jala Neti for the first time may experience some uncomfortable burning sensation in the head, which will disappear after repeated practise of this exercise. This may be done everyday in the early morning. Advanced students of Yoga may perform this with milk or ghee in place of water.

This is one of the easiest of all the Shat Karma practices ensuring profound benefits.

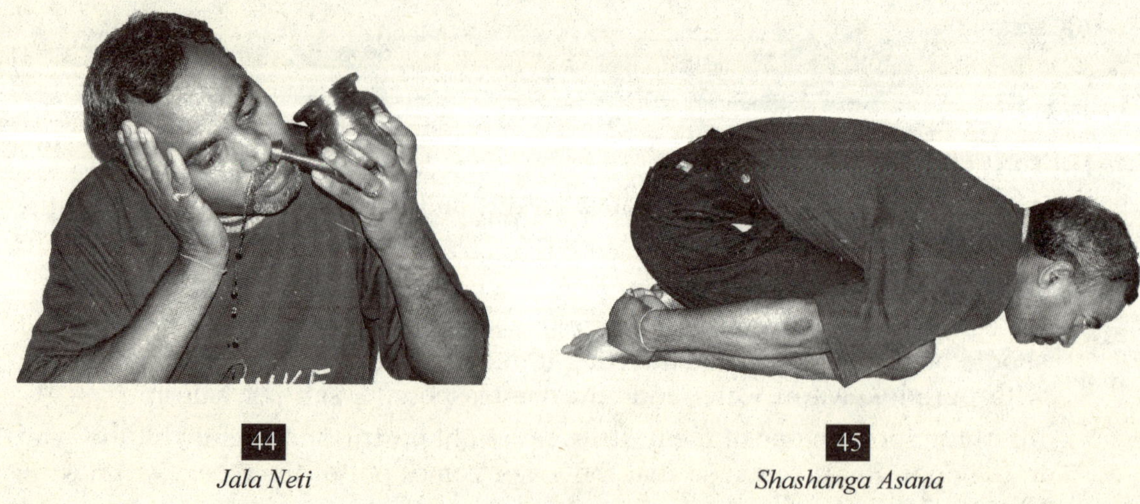

44
Jala Neti

45
Shashanga Asana

Benefits

- ❑ Ensures relief from cold, sinusitis and other disorders of ears, eyes and throat.
- ❑ Chronic headache can be cured.
- ❑ Hair fall and premature greying is arrested.
- ❑ Brings relief to those suffering from insomnia and drowsiness.
- ❑ Particularly good for improving eyesight.
- ❑ The intellect is stimulated by the cooling and soothing effect on the brain.
- ❑ All diseases connected with different organs from the neck upwards can be effectively prevented and cured with the help of Jala Neti.

This exercise is prohibited for those who suffer from chronic haemorrhage in the nose.

(b) Sutra Neti (Cleansing with Thread)

In this exercise, a cotton string of about 20 inches, stiffened with wax, is inserted into one of the nostrils and pulled out from the mouth. Then the string of both sides should be pulled to and fro about 25 to 30 times. Next, insert the cotton string into the other nostril and repeat the same process.

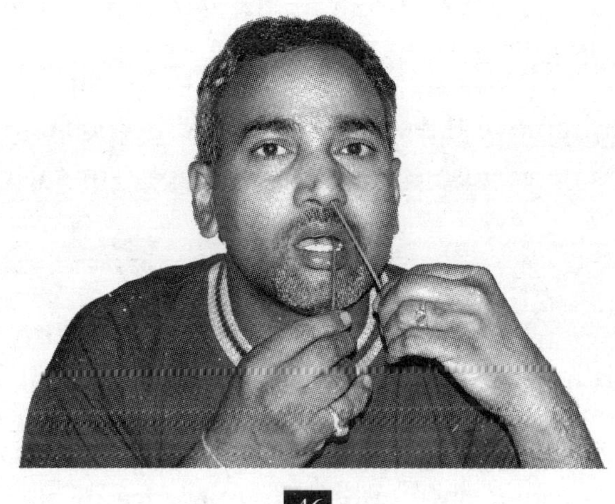

16

Sutra Neti

At times, cotton strings stiffened with wax may not be available. In this case, a thin rubber catherer may be used. This will be available at all leading medical stores.

Jala Neti may be practised after Sutra Neti so that nose blockage may be removed.

This should be attempted only under the guidance of an expert. Those doing this for the first time may experience pain while inserting the string into the nostril. They may also have a sneezing bout in the beginning. This is overcome after repeated practise.

All benefits derived from Jala Neti can also be obtained from Sutra Neti.

2. DHAUTI

(a) Kunjala or Gajakarni

A reference has been made about this exercise in *Bhaktisagara Grantha* as follows:

"What is known as Gajakarni and what makes the body immune to all diseases is filling the stomach with water and bringing it up effortlessly. Just as an elephant draws in water through his trunk, and brings it out through the trunk, thus keeping his body free from all ailments, so can man keep his body free from all sorts of maladies. We clean a pot with the help of water; we clean our stomach with the help of warm water."

As with Jala Neti, keep a vessel filled with warm water mixed with salt of one teaspoon to half a litre proportion. For this exercise, keep at least five to six litres of water.

Sit in a squatting position and drink water as slowly as possible but in quick succession. Continue to drink as many glasses as possible until a vomiting sensation develops. Normally a person can drink five to seven glasses of water at a stretch without any difficulty.

After drinking the water, stand erect and bend forward at an angle of 90 degrees. Keep the left hand on the stomach and with the index and middle fingers of the right hand tickle the uvula situated in the mouth. This will give you a feeling of vomiting and then the water will start coming up in a constant stream. After the flow stops, again tickle the uvula with the fingers and bring up the remaining water. This process should continue until certain that there is no more water inside.

It is necessary that the water should be brought out only in the half-bent posture. It would be harmful to remove the water in a standing position.

This exercise should be performed only on an empty stomach and preferably before dawn.

Benefits

The benefits conferred by this exercise are many. It cures most diseases connected with the stomach, like constipation, indigestion and biliousness. It brings great relief to asthmatic patients. They should form a habit of doing this exercise almost daily so that, in course of time, they will be completely relieved of this disease.

This should be performed only under the guidance of an expert.

Heart patients and persons with high blood pressure should not attempt this without expert guidance.

(b) Vastra Dhauti

The *Hathayogapradipika* (11:24) states: *"One should swallow slowly, as advised by the guru, a wet piece of cloth four fingers (three inches) in breadth and fifteen cubits long, and then draw it out. This process is known as Dhauti."*

This exercise is mainly intended to remove mucus and other waste products from the oesophagus (the gullet) and the stomach. This practice is explained below.

- Secure a fine piece of muslin cloth, three to four inches wide and 15 feet long. It should be ensured that no pieces of loose thread hang from the sides, for which the borders should be well stitched. The cloth should be washed in soap before use and dipped in salt water.
- Sit in a squatting position. Put one end of the cloth in the mouth and swallow it slowly and carefully, mixing it with saliva as one swallows food. On the first day, swallow only one foot of the cloth. This should be kept for a few seconds and then taken out very slowly. On the next day, swallow a little more, and in due course of consistent practice, one would be able to swallow the whole length.
- Beginners should remove the cloth after it is retained for a few minutes. Advanced practitioners can do Nauli exercise after the cloth is inserted into the stomach.

This should never be attempted without the guidance of an expert teacher.

This should be done on an empty stomach, preferably in the morning.

It is always better to leave out at least eight inches of the cloth to enable one to pull out the inserted cloth without any difficulty. In case the cloth does not come out, drink as much water as possible and pull the cloth out by bending forward at the waist and the entire cloth will emerge without difficulty.

The benefits of the exercise are extolled by several authorities on Yoga. The *Hathayogapradipika* (11:25) states: *"As a result of performing Dhauti, asthma, diseases of the spleen and the skin and the 20 varieties of disease caused by phlegm undoubtedly get cured."*

The *Grenda Samitha* (1:42) states: *"With the help of this exercise man can get rid of maladies of the spleen, glandular enlargement in the stomach, fever, cough, bile and leprosy. He becomes strong and healthy."*

(c) Varisara Dhauti or Shankha Prakshalana

This is one of the most important exercises in Shat Karma. There is a lengthy procedure to be followed meticulously. **The guidance of an expert is very essential**, otherwise the practitioner may get into difficulties in performing this accurately. The main purpose of this exercise is to completely wash the alimentary canal from the mouth to the anus with warm alkaline water.

This exercise is to be practised in the early morning on an empty stomach. Even tea, coffee or milk should not be taken before its commencement.

Take a clean plastic bucket or any other similar container filled with warm water mixed with salt. Two teaspoons of salt may be added per litre of water. The temperature of the water should be a few degrees warmer than that for the Kunjala exercise.

Assume the squatting position and drink two glasses of water from the bucket. Then repeat the following four Asanas in quick succession.

(a) Sarpa Asana (Serpent Posture)
(b) Urdhwa Hastottan Asana (Turning Right and Left Posture)
(c) Kati Chakra Asana (Waist Rotating Posture)
(d) Udarakarasa Asana (Abdominal Massage Posture)

(a) Sarpa Asana

- Assume the position of Bhujanga Asana. **(Picture 7)**
- Twist the head towards the right side and gaze at the heel of the opposite foot. **(Picture 47)**
- Repeat the same in the opposite direction. **(Picture 48)**

Perform this four times to the right and four times to the left alternately.

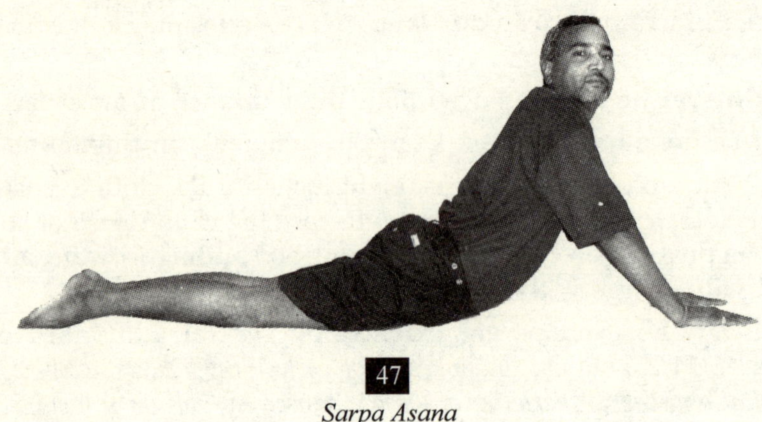

47
Sarpa Asana

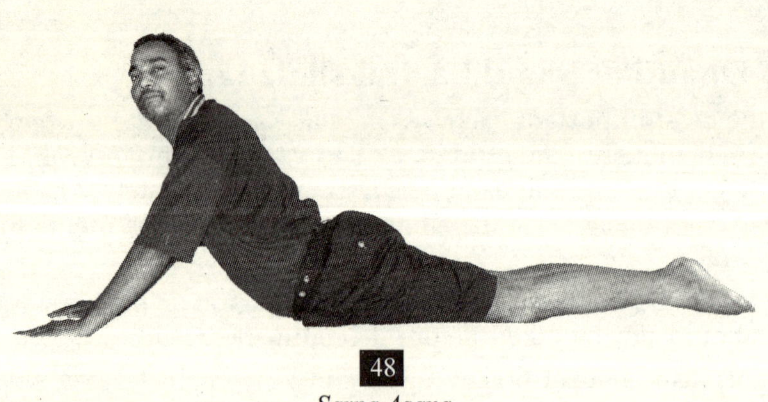

48
Sarpa Asana

(b) Urdhwa Hastottan Asana

- Stand erect.
- Interlock hands and raise them.
- Bend the body towards right making a twist of the stomach. **(Picture 49)**

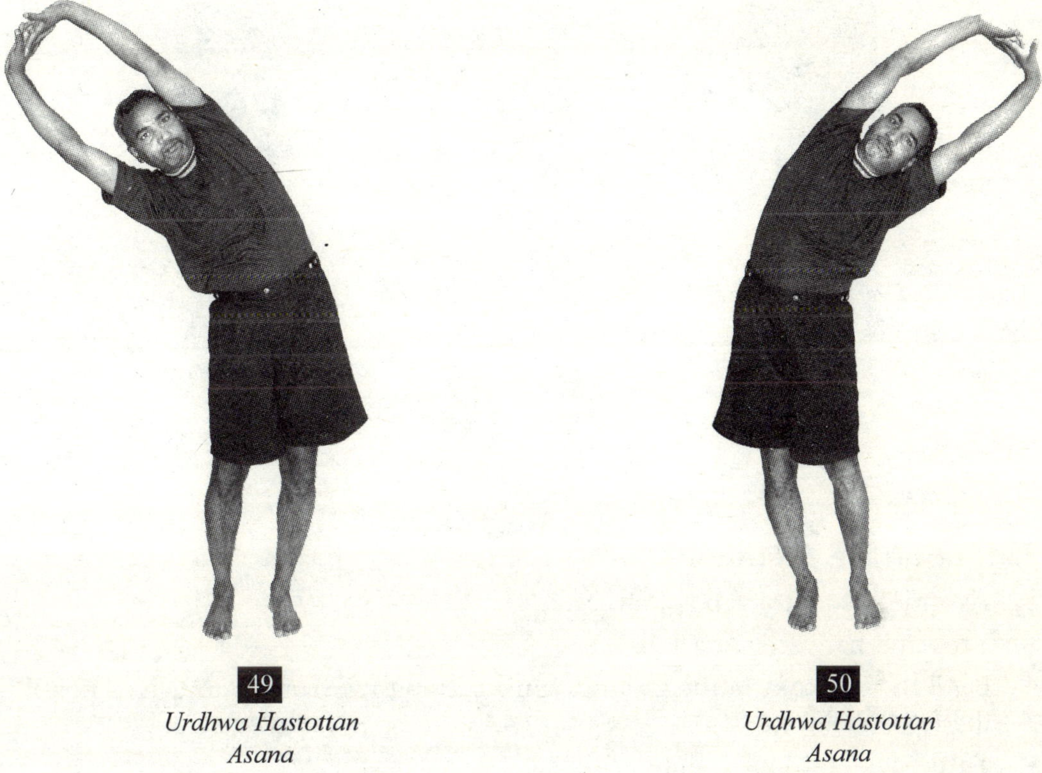

49
Urdhwa Hastottan Asana

50
Urdhwa Hastottan Asana

- Next bend the body towards the left. **(Picture 50)**
- Repeat this four times to the right and four times to the left alternately.

(c) Kati Chakra Asana

- Stand erect keeping the feet about two feet apart.
- Stretch the arms sideways at shoulder level.
- Twist the upper part of the body to the left, bringing the right hand to the left shoulder. **(Picture 51)**
- There should be a twist at the abdomen towards the left.
- Repeat the same towards the right side. **(Picture 52)**
- Continue this alternately four times to the right and four times to the left.

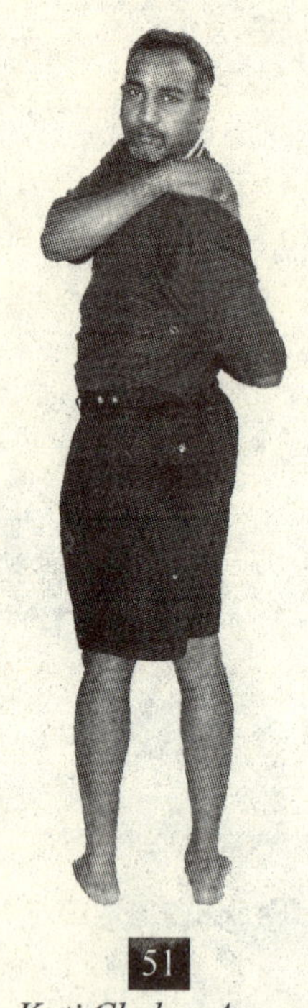

51

Kati Chakra Asana

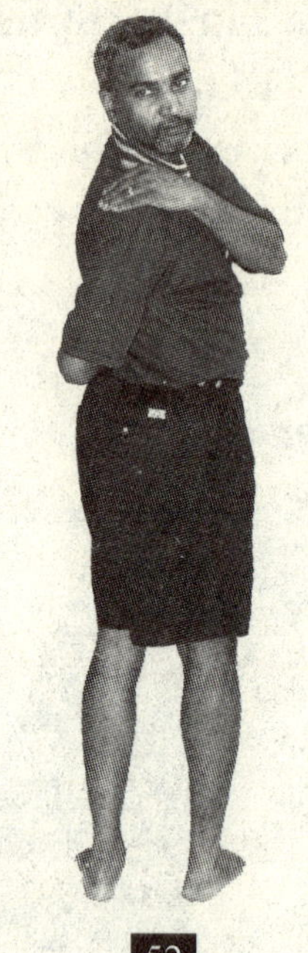

52

Kati Chakra Asana

(d) Udarakarasa Asana

- Assume a squatting position.
- Keep the hands on the knees.
- Bend the left knee to the ground while turning the trunk as much as possible to the left. **(Picture 53)**
- Turn back and look behind.
- Return to the squatting position.
- Repeat the same procedure twisting the body in the opposite direction. **(Picture 54)**
- Repeat this process four times to the right and four times to the left.
- After completing one round of all these four Asanas eight times each, drink two more glasses of water and again perform the four Asanas in the same manner.
- This procedure should be repeated until one feels the sensation to evacuate the bowels. Once this feeling develops, go to the toilet and ease yourself.
- After this, drink two more glasses of water and repeat the Asanas and again visit the toilet.

In this exercise, the stools that come first will be solid, then semi-solid and, finally, of yellowish water.

The process of drinking water and doing the Asanas should be continued along with passing frequent motions until crystal clear water emerges from the bowels.

Before clean water is evacuated one would generally consume 10 to 15 glasses of water on an average. In some special cases of diseased persons, they consume about 25 to 30 glasses of water before crystal clear water is expelled.

After completion of this, drink four or five glasses of lukewarm water with salt and perform Gajakarni and Jala Neti.

Gajakarni cleans the region from the stomach to the mouth and also removes any residue salty water from the stomach. Jala Neti cleans the nasal passages.

After this only warm water bath may be taken. Cold water bath should not be taken after Sankha Prakshalana. A specially prepared meal with rice, ghee and pulse (*mung dal*) should be taken within an hour of completing the exercises.

On this day, the stomach should not be stuffed with heavy meals. Further, for another week it is better to avoid all rich, acidic, chemically processed and non-vegetarian foods.

This may be practised by healthy persons once in six months. For diseased people, the frequency may be changed as per the suggestions of the expert treating the patient through Yogic therapy.

Since this exercise ensures thorough cleaning and irrigation of the entire digestive tract, the benefits accrued from this are innumerable.

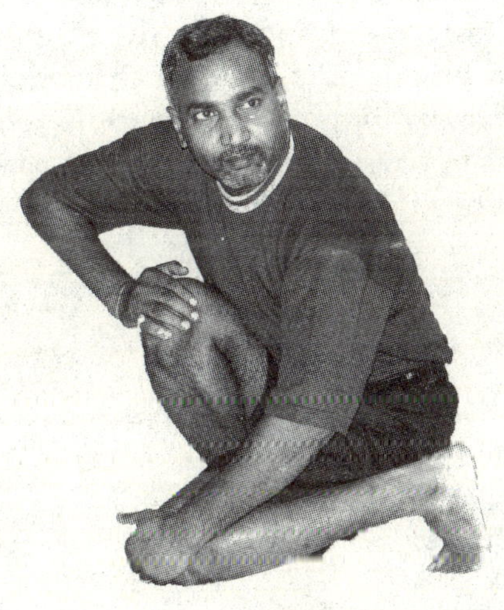

53

Udarakarasa Asana

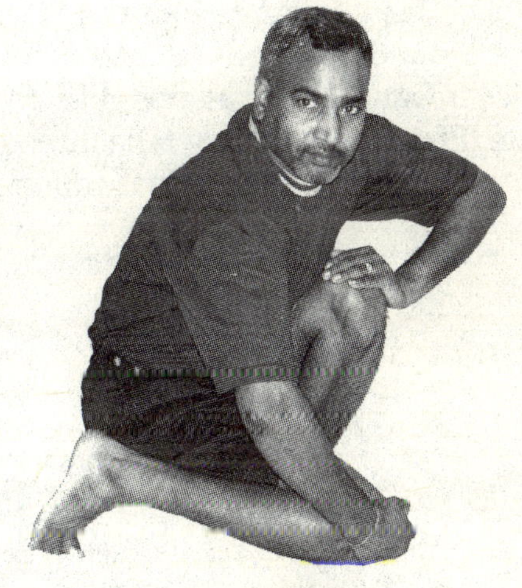

54

Udarakarasa Asana

Benefits

- Cures all diseases connected with the digestive organs. Chronic headaches, diseases of the eyes, nose and teeth are cured.
- Women derive wonderful benefits. Menstrual disorders and barrenness can be cured. It is one of the best exercises for kidney and urinary system and it also helps prevent urinary infections and the formation of kidney stones.

3. BASTI

In this exercise, water is drawn into the bowels through the anus and then expelled.

This can be accomplished quite easily in a flowing river. The manner in which it is practised has been stated in the *Hathayogapradipika* (11:27): *"Adopting the Utkato Asana pose in water coming up to the navel and inserting a tube into the anus, one should contract the anus and wash the interior. This process is known as Basti."*

While standing in the water it is necessary to perform Uddiyana Bandha and Nauli via which the water enters the bowels and also churns the bowels in such a way that the water gets mixed with stools and cleans the bowels thoroughly. The exercise should be repeated four to five times. After this, perform Mayur Asana so that the residue water, stools and wind are removed completely.

The benefits of the exercise have been explained in the *Hathayogapradipika* (11:28) as follows: *"This exercise completely eradicates maladies like abnormal growth in the abdomen, spleen, liver, diseases of the eyes, 25 kinds of urethral irregularities, dyspepsia, constipation, piles, fistula, pimples, boils, acidity, irregularities of the bowels, etc."*

4. NAULI

It is possible to perform this exercise only when one is able to do **Uddiyana Bandha** perfectly. This is done as follows: Stand with legs apart. Bend and hold the thighs with the corresponding hands. Exhale deeply and retain breath outside. Pull up abdominal muscles inward, as far as possible. Maintain this lock as long as the breath is retained outside **(Picture 55)**. It may take three to four months of consistent practise to master this exercise, as various abdominal muscles have to be brought under control.

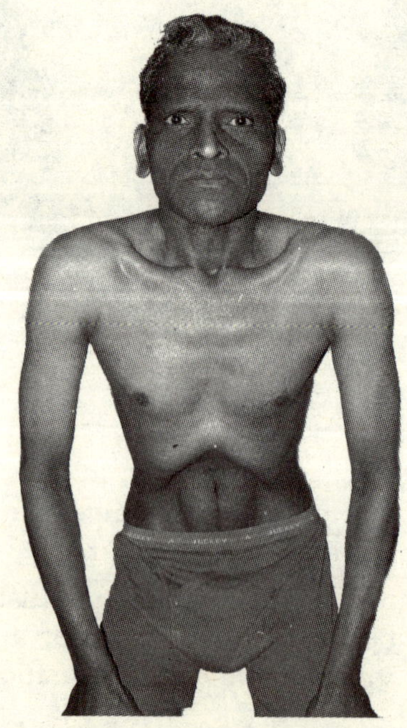

55

Uddiyana Bandha

The main purpose of doing Nauli is to regenerate, invigorate and stimulate the abdominal viscera and the gastrointestinal or alimentary system.

The technique of doing this exercise is as follows:

Madhya Nauli

- Stand with feet separated about two feet.
- Slowly bend and keep the hands on the knees.
- Exhale completely and do Uddiyana Bandha.
- Gently press the arms and draw up the abdominal muscles, focusing your attention on forcing the rectus abdominis to stand out in isolation. This is Madhya Nauli. **(Picture 56)**
- It may not be possible to bring the rectus abdominis to the centre in the initial attempt itself. However, you will succeed with repeated practise.

Vamana Nauli

After successfully manipulating the rectus abdominis to stand out, isolate it on the left side of the abdomen. This is called Vamana Nauli. **(Picture 57)**

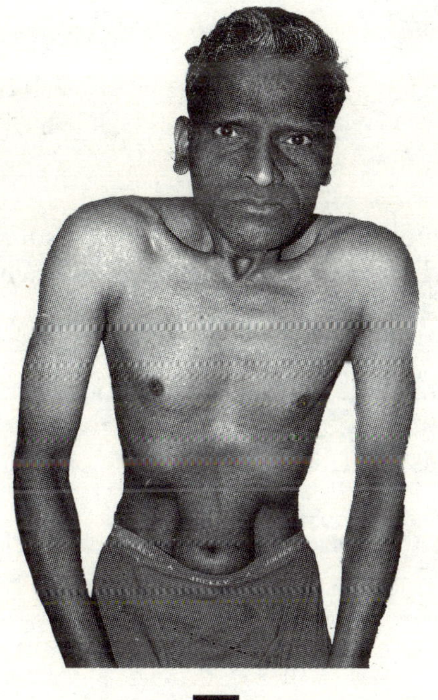

56

Madhya Nauli

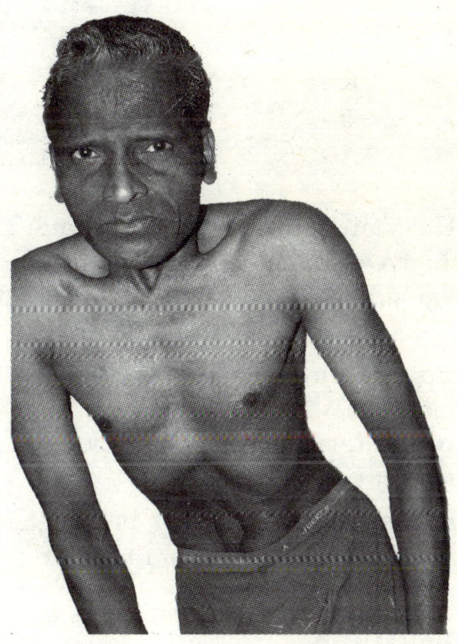

57

Vamana Nauli

Dakshina Nauli

Similarly, the rectus abdominis should be isolated to the right side of the abdomen. This is known as Dakshina Nauli. **(Picture 58)**

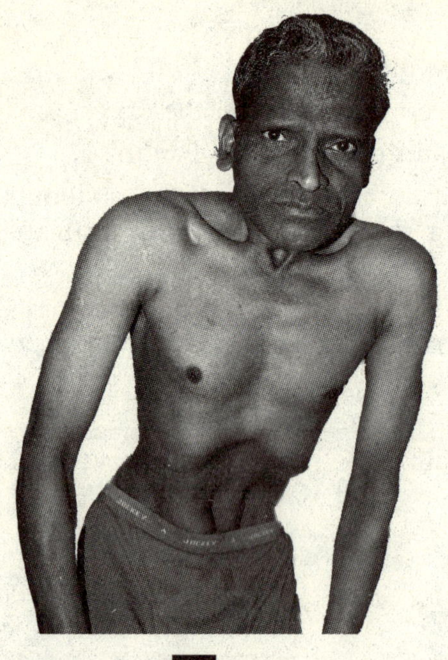

58
Dakshina Nauli

The Vamana and Dakshina Nauli can be performed by applying more pressure on the thighs with the hand. By pressing the left thigh, the rectus abdomini moves towards the left side and the same method applies to the right side also.

After learning to isolate the rectus abdominis to the left and right sides, make an attempt to churn or roll it from the left to the centre and then to the right in one smooth motion. Similarly, the rectus abdominis muscles should be rolled from the right to the centre and then to the left in quick succession. Do this churning exercise for six to eight rounds on each side.

This should necessarily be practised only on an empty stomach, and **under the guidance of an expert yoga teacher**.

Precautions

Persons suffering from high blood pressure, peptic ulcers, hernia and any other serious digestive ailments should not practise this exercise.

Benefits

- Prevents all abdominal ailments.

- Eliminates constipation by encouraging intestinal peristalsis. Keeps sexual organs in good condition and prevents sexual disorders.

Sarvanga Pavana Muktan Kriya (Gas Relief Shoulder Stand)

This is a Kriya, not an Asana. In an Asana one maintains a particular posture for a period of time; in a Kriya, an action has to be performed. Nauli, for example, is a Kriya. In Sarvanga Pavana Muktan Kriya, gas is ejected from the stomach many times.

Technique

- Do Sarvanga Asana. **(Picture 21)**
- Bring both legs down close to the forehead. The legs should be slightly separated and loosely hung.
- Breathe out and do Madhya Nauli.
- Press the rectus abdominis up and down in such a way that the gas in the stomach is ejected. If Nauli Kriya is mastered, it is possible to eject gas even 50 to 60 times, depending upon the amount of gas formed in the stomach. **(Picture 59)**

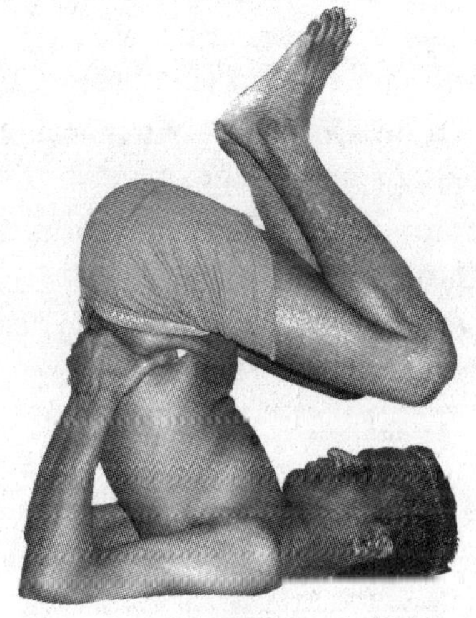

59
Sarvanga Pavana
Muktan Asana

Sarvanga Pavana Muktan Kriya may be done immediately after Mayura Asana. In Mayura Asana, the abdomen is greatly compressed and accumulated gas starts rushing out when this Kriya is done correctly.

5. KAPALABHATI

One of the Pranayama exercises described under Pranayama No. 3.

6. TRATAKA

An exercise mainly intended to improve eyesight and the power of concentration via the technique of gazing at one point. There are different techniques available for this purpose, but the one advocated by Yogis is to use a lighted candle. This is practised as follows:

Sit in one of the meditative postures, preferably in Padma Asana. Keep a lighted candle two to three feet away at the level of the eyes. The spine should be kept erect but the whole body should be relaxed. Gaze intently at the brightest part of the flame without making any movement of the eyes or blinking. This should be continued until the eyes are tired and begin to water. Then close your eyes and relax. Even after closing the eyes the after-image of the candle flame must be visualised till the image fades and goes out of consciousness. Then open the eyes and repeat the procedure for 10 to 15 minutes.

After consistent practise for a few months, one will find that many minor lights surround the flaming spot.

Efforts should be made to ensure there is no deflection from the central spot. One is said to have succeeded in the practise of Trataka only when one sees nothing but light in the direction in which one looks at.

Another form of this exercise is to concentrate and focus the eyes on the eyebrow centre. This is known as Shambhavi Mudra (Eyebrow Centre Gazing). (**Picture 61**)

Trataka can also be practised on any object, such as a small dot on the wall, the nose tip, the statue of a saint, a cross or any other object of choice.

The eyes should not be strained too much. The duration of keeping the eyes open and gazing at the lit candle or any other object should be developed gradually over time.

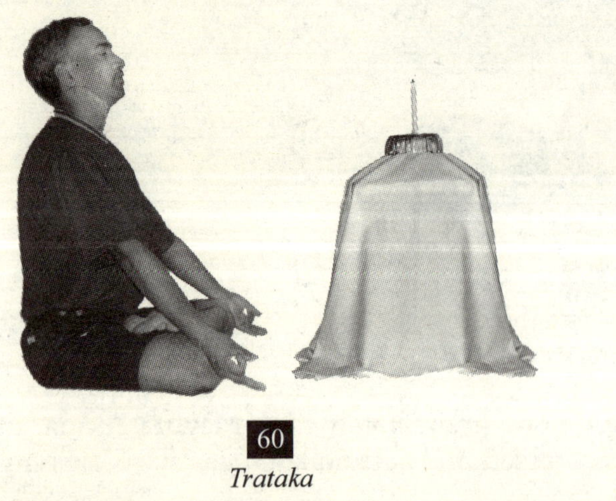

60

Trataka

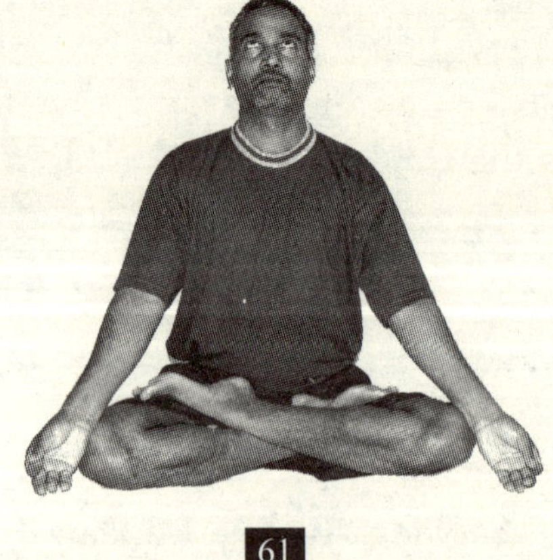

61

Shambhavi Mudra
(Eyebrow centre gazing)

Benefits

Strengthens muscles of the eyes and corrects defects like night blindness, short-sightedness, etc. Develops the power of concentration, calms the mind and removes stress and strain.

Part Five

Theory and Practise of Meditation

Introduction

A king, noted for his egoistic tendency, conquered many countries. He was able to command anything he wanted in the materialistic realm. But most of the time, he felt a vacuum inside his heart. He did not have peace of mind and happiness in his life. He had killed many people in war. He was always tormented by the fact whether he would go to Heaven or Hell after death. He tried all possible means to gain peace of mind, but in vain.

Then one of his ministers suggested he seek the advice of a renowned Buddhist monk living in the jungle. The king went to meet the monk with his entourage. At this time the monk was in deep meditation. The king waited for quite some time.

Unfortunately, the monk did not emerge from his meditative trance. The king no longer had the patience to wait anymore and he physically shook the monk. The monk's meditation was disturbed.

At this point, the king asked the monk: "Which is the way to go to Heaven or Hell?"

The monk opened his eyes, looked at him sternly and said: "Foolish man! Don't you have any sense? You have disturbed my meditation."

Hearing this, the king was terribly upset and felt very insulted. Angrily, he drew his sword to kill the monk. Unmoved by the king's action, the monk smilingly said: "This is the way to go to Hell."

Seeing the smiling face of the monk, the king immediately understood that the monk was not really angry with him but had spoken with some inner meaning. He came to his senses, withdrew the sword, and asked for pardon.

Now, the monk said: "This is the way to Heaven."

The king was surprised at the wisdom of the monk and asked politely: "I have conquered many countries. But I have no peace of mind. What should I do to gain peace and happiness in life?"

To this, the monk replied: "When I die you shall gain peace and happiness."

The king could not comprehend this and asked, "Why should you die for my peace of mind."

At this, the monk told him: "You have misunderstood my statement. What I meant by the word 'I' is your egoistic tendency. Only when your ego dies will you develop humility and the virtue of humility will provide you the happiness you seek."

All saints, seers and sages regularly practise meditation with the sole objective of obliterating their ego. They are the embodiment of humility. This virtue can be developed through meditation.

If you keenly observe the functioning of your mind, you will notice that you are talking to yourself. Most of the self-talk revolves around your personal problems. It could be your family or profession, your happiness and achievements, your problems and sufferings, etc. Your consciousness, which is a stream of thoughts and feelings, is totally saturated with personal problems. As long as you entertain thoughts relating to personal problems and difficulties, you experience greater stress in life. One of the ways to overcome stress is to practise meditation.

Meditation is a process through which one makes an attempt to forget his self through a variety of techniques.

Defining Meditation

Here are some definitions of meditation.

- ME-DIG-ACTION is meditation. You try to understand the inner functioning of your mind.
- Making an inner journey.
- The process of stilling the mind.
- Emptying the mind.
- The negation of self.
- Taking away consciousness from external entanglement.
- An altered state of consciousness.
- Making peace with the inner self.
- Establishing a link between the higher regions of the mind and waking consciousness.
- **Shifting consciousness from the self to something else.**

Benefits of Meditation

- ❑ Brings profound relaxation, both physical and mental. One of the remarkable changes that occur during meditation is slowing down of the metabolic rate – the rate at which the body burns oxygen and food necessary for building up the body.
- ❑ Lowers blood pressure, both during and after meditation.
- ❑ Slows down the heart rate to a few beats per minute.

- Increased blood flow ensures that oxygen is more efficiently delivered to the muscles and the lactate produced during periods of intensive activity is more quickly and effectively removed.
- Calmness and serenity ensure the production of lactate is less. Conversely, those experiencing anxiety, tension and neurosis have a high level of lactate.
- With reduction in lactate level during meditation, deep relaxation is experienced, which consequently reduces blood pressure and all anxiety symptoms.
- Regular practise brings about an improvement in psychosomatic diseases.
- Practitioners show increased intelligence, memory, emotional stability, personality strengths and an enormous improvement in social and vocational adjustments, because meditation imparts mental discipline.

The person who meditates becomes physiologically better from the person who does not. Physiologically meditation is deeply restful, much more than the normal rest gained from lying on a cosy bed in deep sleep.

Regular practise of meditation transforms a person gradually by imparting a sense of calm and control. Transformation does not take place during sleep although the body gains physical relaxation. Meditation paves the way for spiritual growth. Meditation ensures inner peace and harmony.

The emotional turmoil of daily life is neutralised by deep meditation. During meditation, one will notice the remarkable improvements that occur in the brain rhythm, blood pressure, pulse rate, skin resistance, etc.

In recent years, scientists have begun to notice the profound impact of meditation in curing many so-called incurable diseases. Dr Carl Simonton from the United States has cured several terminal cancer patients through his CRVR meditation technique.

Practising Meditation

There are many techniques for meditation. Only a few are presented here. They are easy to practise but powerful and effective in managing stress and in improving one's health and personality. These are:

1. Simple Meditation
2. Chitta Meditation
3. Baghya Kumbaka Meditation
4. Sabdha Meditation
5. Vipassana Meditation
6. Soham Meditation
7. Zen Meditation
8. Trataka Meditation
9. Transcendental Meditation
10. Christian Meditation

11. Yogic Chakra Meditation
12. Jnana Yoga Meditation
13. Subconscious Meditation
14. Creative Dynamic Meditation
15. CRVR Meditation
16. Digital Meditation

1. Simple Meditation

Technique

Sit in a meditative posture, Sukha Asana **(Picture 62)** or Padma Asana **(Picture 63)**, forming Jnana Mudra and with the eyes closed.

Stay in this posture for about 15 minutes, making your subconscious believe that you are meditating. There is no specific technique given here. The main purpose is to acquaint you with self-discipline to be able to sit quietly for a given length of time. This is a preliminary step for the practise of other types of meditation.

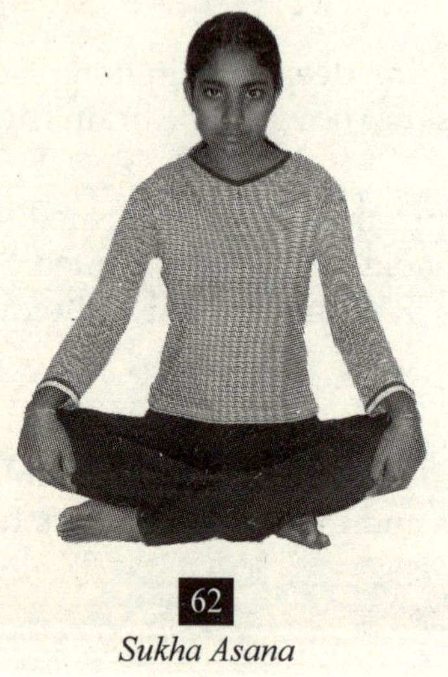

62
Sukha Asana

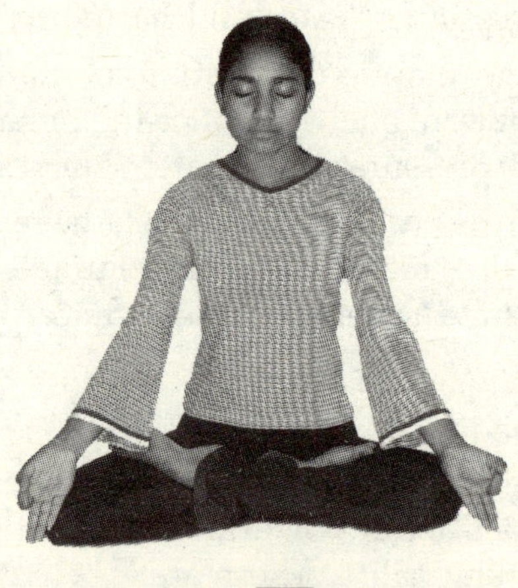

63
Padma Asana

Special Remarks

Parents wishing to teach their children self-discipline may adopt this technique by making the children simply sit for a specific length of time, preferably in Padma Asana. Discipline means creating order within you.

2. Chitta Meditation (Consciousness Meditation)

Technique

Sit in a meditative posture, forming Jnana Mudra and with the eyes closed **(Picture 63)**. Keep calm and quiet and observe your thoughts and feelings.

Do not attempt either to control or direct your thoughts. Act only as an objective observer of each thought, feeling, perception, etc. that is being screened on your mental horizon. When a thought or feeling arises, simply observe it until it passes out of your visual space. Then you may wait for the next thought or feeling and observe it till it remains. Do not make any attempt to explore, follow up or associate with any thoughts or feelings passing through your mind.

Observing personal thoughts or feelings without getting involved may appear paradoxical. But practise makes you perfect. Try this meditation for a week consistently without any break and you may find it quite practical.

Do not be perturbed if the same thought or feeling arises repeatedly.

If your mind goes "blank", continue in this state for as long as possible. This is a good indication that you are on the right path.

Special Remarks

Chitta means *consciousness* and refers to the stream of thoughts and feelings. Its main intent is to understand the process of our thoughts and feelings. It is the first step in the attainment of self-realisation. This meditation can be practised in any place and in any posture. The moment you are aware of your thoughts and feelings, you are in a meditative state. I strongly suggest that everyone should start practising this meditation technique. It is simple and very effective.

3. Bhakya Kumbaka Meditation

Bhakya Kumbaka denotes outer retention. This technique is meant to fully relax body and mind.

When we inhale we bring Prana (life energy) into the body. This gives strength to the body and keeps it in good condition. When we exhale, the chest is constricted and pure blood is pumped from the heart to the rest of the body. With the flow of fresh blood the whole body is refreshed and replenished. The body thus gets energy while inhaling and relaxes after exhalation.

Between exhalation and inhalation there is a pause. This is the pause of relaxation. The present meditation technique is based on this principle.

Technique

Sit relaxed in any posture or lie down.

Inhale deeply, and without pause exhale slowly and deeply.

After exhalation, maintain outer retention for about ten seconds or for as long as you feel comfortable holding your breath. During this pause mentally repeat the word RELAX five or ten times. Then inhale.

Benefits

Fifteen minutes of this meditation will give you the kind of relaxation you may not have experienced all your life. This is one of the most efficacious techniques to secure relief from tension, stress and anxiety.

4. Sabdha Meditation

Sabdha means *sound*. Meditation does not necessarily need a secluded, calm and quiet place. It can be practised even in a moving bus or train. Travel confines you to a particular spot and can be the best opportunity for meditation.

External distractions do not matter. Meditation requires that you take your mind off the humdrum of daily life and concentrate on only one thing at a time.

Technique

The drone of the moving bus or the chug-chugging of the train itself could be the object of meditation. Concentrate your whole attention on the sound. When your mind slips off, bring it back and be aware of the sound only and nothing else.

Incidentally, you may realise that the excuse that you do not have time for meditation does not hold water. This technique is another instance where you can meditate under most circumstances.

5. Vipassana Meditation

Technique

Vipassana refers to the breathing process. This meditation can be practised in any place or in any posture. Your own breathing process forms the focus of attention here. Breathing is an unconscious act and does not warrant our conscious effort.

In this technique, an attempt should be made to direct our consciousness towards our breathing only. When some other thought intrudes, push them aside. This is the first step to control our thoughts through the process of breathing.

6. Soham Meditation

Soham is one of the mantras. A mantra is a word specially used by Indian Yogis to bring some beneficial results to humanity at large when repeated mentally or orally. Mantras need not have any specific meaning as such. The Vedas state that the word ***Soham*** has special significance to produce peace and tranquillity.

Technique

Bring your total attention on breathing as you have done in Vipassana meditation. Instead of merely observing your breathing process, mentally repeat the word ***Soham***, synchronising it with your breath.

When you inhale, mentally repeat the sound SO and while exhaling say HAM. As you breathe in and out the sound ***Soham*** should be repeated.

7. Zen Meditation

Is there any possibility of arresting our thought process through physical manipulation? Yes. There is. This technique is called Shambhavi Mudra (Gazing at the Eyebrow Centre). In this technique, one should try to look at the centre of the eyebrow. When a person tries to look at his eyebrow centre, he cannot think. If he tries to think, he may get a mild headache. Zen Meditation has combined Shambhavi Mudra **(Picture 61)** with the awareness of breathing.

Technique

This meditation can be practised in any comfortable and restful posture. Look at the eyebrow centre. At the same time your awareness should be on your breathing. When some other thought intrudes, push them aside. At times, merely concentrating on our breath may be difficult. In order to fix our attention completely on the breathing, you may start counting your breath with every exhalation: one, two, three, etc. All your attention is gently and firmly fixed on this one action of counting only. You may count sequentially, as high as you can go during each session.

Sequential counting has a pitfall – it is very difficult to concentrate. You will be able to count without being aware of it. It becomes an automatic activity and your thoughts may plunge into something unwanted.

To counteract this, the counting may be varied slightly: count up to 50 or even beyond, and then count backwards.

This type of meditation is taught in Zen training, where students are required to be aware of their breathing process all the time.

Since breathing is a continuous unbroken process it provides you the means for unbroken meditation on which you can concentrate non-stop until the expiry of the scheduled time you have set apart for yourself.

If the breathing is rhythmic, a sort of vibration is created in the body, which tones up your nervous system and thereby reduces stress.

8. Trataka Meditation

Technique

Sit in a meditative posture, forming Jnana Mudra, with the eyes closed. Keep an object before you – an idol, a cross, a photo or picture of your role model, etc. Visualise it with closed eyes **(Picture 60)**.

Your thoughts should continuously be saturated on the object of visualisation. When it strays, bring it back and focus attention on the object.

Practise this for 15 minutes daily.

Benefits

Apart from arresting the wavering mind, this meditation will also improve concentration, imagination and eyesight.

9. Transcendental Meditation (TM)

This is one of the several meditative techniques originally innovated by a seer named Shankara who lived 2,500 years ago. The unique contribution of Maharishi Mahesh Yogi lies in making a small modification in the technique so that people of all cultures and social conditions can easily practise it.

Technique

Claudio Naranjo and Robert E Ornstein, authors of the book, *On the Psychology of Meditation*, have explained the technique of TM as follows:

"In this form of meditation (TM) the practitioner is given a specific mantra and he has to repeat it silently over and over for about half-hour twice a day in the morning and in the evening. No special posture is required for the exercise; rather, one is instructed to assume a comfortable posture, such as sitting erect in a chair. The thoughts that arise during the meditation are considered to be of no significance and as soon as one is aware that one is no longer focused on this mantra, attention is to be returned to it.

"The specific mantras used in Transcendental Meditation are not given publicity, since the devotees of this technique claim that there are special effects of each one in addition to the general effects of the concentration. But it can be noted here that these mantras are also mellifluous and smooth, including many M's and Y's and vowels, similar to OM or MU in Zen. Devotees of Transcendental Meditation also claim that this technique involves the essence of meditation in a form suitable for Western persons. There is no doubt Mantra Yoga, including Transcendental Meditation, is a very convenient form of meditation. As in the breathing exercises, it is quite easy to produce and attend to a silent word, any where, at any time. Since there is no special posture required, the arduous training for sitting in a lotus position is unnecessary."

The reasons for the popularity of TM are many. Among the many meditation techniques available, TM is the easiest to learn. It can be practised by all persons irrespective of age, religion, nationality etc. The technique is so simple that anybody can teach it. One of the important qualifications for the instructor of TM is that he should know all the mantras on the basis of individual requirement. It brings profound results to the practitioner in return for the limited effort and time invested.

For the first time in the history of spirituality, research has been conducted extensively on meditation in general and TM in particular and it has been proved that meditation produces wholesome effects on psychological and physiological mechanisms of human beings. Apart from all these, Maharishi Mahesh Yogi is one of the best salesmen among religious teachers, who fully used the mass media of press, radio and television to propagate the usage of TM worldwide.

The positive value of mantras is in the "vibrational" qualities of certain sounds and the effect of these vibrations on specific parts of the body or personality. Mantra sounds are supposed to vibrate in certain organs of the body and stimulate them to function better and also to bring them into greater harmony with other organs and personality areas.

The choice of a mantra is crucial. In India, the Guru (the preceptor) prescribes mantras to his *shisya* (disciple) when initiating him into spiritual life. Mantras are mostly taken from the Vedas.

In ***Meditation from Tantras,*** Swami Satyananda Saraswathi from the Bihar School of Yoga has given some mantras for various religious people and for different purposes. A sampling of these mantras is given here. You may practise Mantra Meditation according to your requirements.

From the Upanishads	:	*Aum, Sivoham (Soham)*
Seed Mantras	:	*Aum, Shrim, Ayim, Ayinga,* etc.
For Removing Disease	:	*Aum Hrim Hansa*
For Sound Health	:	*Achutham Chamritham, Chaiva Japedoushadhkarmani*
For Wealth	:	*Aum Shrim Mahalakshmiyia Namaha*
Sikh Mantra	:	*Sat Nam*
Jain Mantra	:	*Arhint Siddha*
Buddhist Mantra	:	*Buddham Saranam Gachami*
Islamic Mantra	:	*Allahu, Allahu*
Christian Mantra	:	*Ave Maria, Sanctus, Sanctus*

10. Christian Meditation

The aim of meditation is to take consciousness away from external entanglements even for a short time and direct it inwards and ultimately achieve progressively the unfoldment of the practitioner's innate capacities through self-realisation. Through constant practise of meditation one is able to manifest all his potential to the peak and attain perfect harmony with his inner being and his external environment. All types of meditation techniques attempt to achieve this objective.

Christian Meditation differs fundamentally from Yoga Meditation in its approach and content. For Christians, the object of meditation is Christ Himself. The life of Christ, His Passion, His characteristics and His teachings form the main focus of concentration. Christ is the embodiment of love, humility and compassion. He is the Saviour of humanity and He gives heavenly peace and bliss. In Christian Meditation, the practitioner is required to exclusively contemplate on Christ. The idea is that one should emulate the life and character of Christ through repeated practise of meditation. Christian Meditation forms part of another kind of prayer without the aid of rosaries, prayer books and missals. It is an unstructured prayer in which a person establishes direct and personal communication with Christ.

St. Theresa of Avila has advocated a systematic approach to meditation. The following are the five general steps formulated by her to practise meditation.

1. **Preparation:** In the preparatory stage the meditator is required to have complete surrender to God Almighty. Meditation should be approached with all humility for which he should physically feel the presence of Christ with the fond hope that Christ would help him all through the process of meditation. In Christian Meditation there is no question of mind control but the attitude with which the meditation is taken up is very important.
2. **Selection of Material:** Since meditation implies conversations with Christ, one is obliged to select a subject for meditation. This may be preferably taken from the Gospels. St. Theresa states that our meditation period will find us frequently occupied with our Lord, His life and His doctrine.
3. **The Consideration:** After having felt the presence of Christ and with the proper material selected, the meditator should begin to reflect upon the material. In order to make the reflection more effective one may ask oneself certain questions. Who is here in this scene? What is He doing? What does it mean to me? These questions mostly relate to the visualisation of the meditator during the hours of meditation.
4. **The Conversation:** This is the principal part of the meditation. The meditator practically begins the actual conversation with Christ. It should be a heart-to-heart discussion. The meditator is left free to converse on whatever he wants to discuss with Christ. During the course of such a conversation, the meditator affirms his faith in Christ. He may openly express his love for Him and also his desire to serve Him to the best of his ability. The presence of Christ must be physically felt. He may ask His pardon for the wrong done and thank Him for the favours received and also request Him to provide more strength and will-power to withstand the temptations to commit sins and further assure Him about not committing any more sins in the future.
5. **The Conclusion:** During the concluding phase of meditation, the meditator evaluates the extent to which he was able to meditate on Christ and also thanks Him for the guidance He gave during Meditation. Further, he resolves to hold a better and purposeful conversation with Christ in the subsequent period of meditation.

Emotional attachment to Christ is the prerequisite for successful completion of Christian Meditation. Most Christian saints had the experience of reaching the ecstatic state merely by meditating intensely on Christ. These persons experienced supreme joy, happiness and bliss during such an ecstatic state.

11. Yogic Chakra Meditation

Yogic Meditation involves the manipulation of physical and psychological aspects of the human system through certain well-defined techniques and methods. Its ultimate objective is to reach the Samadhi state. In order to reach Samadhi, Yogis perform a series of Yogic practices such as Asanas, Bandhas, Mudras, Shat Karma, concentration and meditation. It is quite easy for a Yogi to reach the Samadhi state once he is fully established in the practices of meditation.

The first step in Yogic Meditation begins with ordinary concentration of the mind on some external object such as gazing at the lighted candle (Trataka), or looking intently at a small dot, a ball, a statue, the tip of the nose (Nasikagra Drishti), eyebrow centre (Shambhavi Mudra) etc., for a considerable period of time. This is done in order to control the wavering mind.

Another form of Yogic Meditation is repeating certain mantras either mentally or vocally. The mental repetition of mantras forms part of Transcendental Meditation, the specific technique of which has already been discussed.

An advanced form of Yogic Meditation is to concentrate on the seven Chakras situated in different parts of the body. These Chakras are associated with major nerve plexuses and endocrinal glands in the body. The entire human system is controlled by these Chakras and they have profound influence on the total personality of individuals. During meditation awareness must be focused on these Chakras.

The particulars of different Chakras with their related importance to the practice of meditation are given below:

1. **Mooladhara Chakra:** Located at the base of the spinal column, it lies between the origin of the reproductory organ and the anus. Its position is the lowest of all the Chakras. It is related to the **earth element** in nature and corresponds to the **Sacro-coccygeal Plexus** in the physical body.

Mooladhara is considered the seat of primal energy known as Kundalini Shakti or sexual energy. This energy can be transformed into potential motive force for the development of physical, mental and psychic powers in man. By meditating intensely on this Chakra, the Yogi is capable of stimulating the Kundalini Shakti, which will begin to rise. When it reaches the next Chakra, i.e. Swadhisthana, the sexual power and energy of the Yogi is very heightened. At this stage, he is expected to control his sexual passion and meditate further on the other charkas. This process should continue until the Kundalini Shakti reaches the last one, Sahasrara, and he attains the state of Samadhi.

2. **Swadhisthana Chakra:** This is located above the Mooladhara Chakra in the spinal region directly behind the genital organ. The corresponding centre in the physical body of the nervous system for this Chakra is the **Prostatic Plexus**. This Chakra is mainly associated with the organs of excretion and reproduction. Meditation on the Chakra will rectify any disorders in these functions. It relates to the **water element** in nature and a person meditating on this Chakra will have no fear of water. Moreover, such persons will get many psychic powers, intuition and a perfect control over the senses.

3. **Manipura Chakra:** This is the third one from the Mooladhara Chakra situated within Sushumna Nadi near the navel region. It has control over digestive organs. Meditation on this Chakra is supposed to increase digestive capacity. This Chakra represents the **fire element** and is associated with vitality and energy. It corresponds to the **Solar Plexus** in the body.

4. **Anahata Chakra:** This is situated near the heart region. It corresponds to the **Cardiac Plexus** in the physical body. Related to the **air element** in nature, it is associated with the heart and lungs and the functions of circulatory and respiratory systems. Practitioners of Yoga should meditate on this Chakra while performing Asanas in order to get relief from diseases connected with the heart and lungs: bronchitis, asthma, tuberculosis, anaemia, hypertension, etc.
5. **Vishuddhi Chakra:** This is located within the Sushumna Nadi at the base of the throat in the region of the Adam's apple. This corresponds to the **Laryngeal Plexus** in the physical body. This Chakra influences the vocal cords and the region of the larynges, thyroid and parathyroid glands. By meditating intently on this Chakra, one can remove disorders in this area of the physical body. It relates to the **ether element** in nature.
6. **Ajna Chakra:** This is also situated within the Sushumna Nadi at the space between the eyebrows. The corresponding centre in the physical body is the **Cavernous Plexus**. This Chakra is a well-known centre used for concentration in many systems of meditation. For concentration, the eyebrow centre is selected, but the real seat of Ajna Chakra is within the area of the brain. Its corresponding physical part is the pineal gland, a tiny pea-sized gland within the brain. On the psychic plane this delicate point is the **bridge between the physical, mental and psychic bodies**. By meditating on this Chakra, one can develop supramental faculties, such as clairvoyance, clairaudience, telepathy and other abilities that lie latent in every human being.
7. **Sahasrara:** This is not considered a Chakra but supposed to **contain all the other Chakras** within itself. It is the **abode of the highest consciousness**. The five lower Chakras are related to finer elements progressing up to the Ajna Chakra, which is the subtlest. Mooladhara – earth, the grossest element in nature; Swadhisthana – water, less grosser than earth; Manipura – fire, subtler than water; Anahata – air, subtler than fire; Vishuddhi – ether, subtler than the rest. **Ajna – the subtlest of all the five elements of nature represents consciousness.** The five elements of nature assigned to the first five Chakras and consciousness representing the Ajna Chakra and Sahasrara are only **symbolic** and the real significance is that through constant meditational practices the Yogi is expected to **transcend his personality from the grossest manifestation of worldly desires, passions and instincts to that of the subtlest one of intuition, inspiration, creativity and bliss** constituting the way to **spiritual emancipation**.

It was stated earlier that Mooladhara Chakra is the seat of Kundalini Shakti. One of the aims of the practice of Yogic Meditation is to awaken this Kundalini Shakti through **self-purification and concentration** of mind on various Chakras referred to above. When the Yogi succeeds in his meditational practices, Kundalini Shakti, the primal energy in man, moves upward through all the other Chakras, step by step, according to the duration and intensity of meditation, and then **reaches the topmost** one, Sahasrara. At this stage, the Yogi attains **Samadhi** and experiences supreme **joy, happiness and bliss**.

12. Jnana Yoga Meditation

Jnana means *wisdom*. The purpose of this meditation is to get enlightened. The technique adopted here is not to concentrate on an object or sound but to reflect on a series of queries posed by the meditator himself. The nature of the questions are such that he may not be able to find answers for all. However, he is expected to think over them seriously.

No special posture is required and this can also be practised in all places, at any time and in any posture.

The questions generally posed in this meditation are:

- Who am I?
- Am I the body?
- Am I the mind?
- Am I the body and mind?
- Where have I come from?
- What was I before my birth?
- Who is responsible for my birth?
- Why was I born in this country?
- Why not in some other country?
- What will happen to me tomorrow?
- Can I predict my future?
- Can I decide the number of children I should have?
- How many male?
- How many female?
- Is it in my control?
- How long will I live?
- Can I avoid death?
- Can I postpone old age and death?
- Can I decide my own longevity?
- What will happen to me after death?
- Is there any life after death?
- Will I be born again?
- How big is this earth?
- How big is this universe?
- Is it not a fact that there are innumerable stars and suns in this universe?
- How big am I in this universe?
- Am I not just a drop in the ocean?
- How many were born before me?
- How many are living in the present?

- How many will be born in future?
- Am I not one among the billions and billions of people who inherited this earth?
- Still, don't I feel that I am great? Superior? Wonderful? Efficient?
- Am I not an atom of atoms when compared to the magnitude of this universe?
- Don't I feel proud of myself?
- Why should I have such egotism?
- Is it not good to be humble?
- Will not humility bring me peace of mind?

Ask as many questions as possible and of all varieties. There is no necessity to have any order in these questions. The more we ask the more we get enlightened on so many things. When we look at things from the broader perspective of the universe, we are **greatly humbled**. This will definitely bring us **peace of mind**.

All problems of humanity at large emerge from the fact that everyone thinks he is superior to others in one way or the another.

This meditation technique will make the meditator more realistic and pragmatic in his approach to the problems of life. This will also **pave the way for spiritual awareness**.

13. Subconscious Meditation

Technique

The technique is simple. You have to saturate your mind with beautiful, inspiring and idealistic thoughts. Write down the things you want as slogans and during meditation run these slogans through your mind, letting their full import and meaning lodge within your subconscious. Quotes of eminent persons are useful.

To Develop Confidence

When you feel diffident and lack confidence and courage, it may help to repeat over and over again in the hours of meditation the following quote from Swami Vivekananda.

"Have faith that you are all, my brave lad, born to do great things. Let not the barks of puppies frighten you: no, not even the thunderbolts of heaven, but stand up and work."

To Attain Serenity

Many things occur in life that are beyond our control and comprehension. They are inevitable in everyday life and need to be accepted humbly. When faced with unavoidable sorrows, it may help to meditate on this verse of Reinhold Niebuhr:

"God, grant me the serenity

To accept the things I cannot change;

The courage to change the things I can

And the wisdom to know the difference."

Surrender to God

Sorrow is also sublimated when placed in the perspective of the sorrows of the wider world. A meditation using the following affirmation of Edgar Cayce will help in placing this in perspective:

"Not my way, Lord. Have thine own way with me."

Ensuring Peaceful Sleep

An insomniac could invite refreshing sleep by meditating. Just before going to sleep recall the words of Norvell:

"I shall now fall into deep, natural and refreshing sleep. My mind is still and peaceful as a lake in the midst of a silent forest at midnight. I am surrounded by a sea of calmness. My mind is now retreating through the corridors of time back into timelessness. I am once again a child, without worries or cares on my mind. I have faith that God will protect me and solve all my problems, I am now floating on a cloud, up... up... up... into realms of forgetfulness, peace and beauty. I now sleep, sleep, sleep."

You may construct your own statement to suit your requirement and use it during meditation. The statement should be crisp, effective and, if possible rhythmic, so that when it is repeated mentally over and over again, vibrations will be generated in the body.

Instead of sentences and verses, only one word may also be chosen for this purpose. The word may be repeated a hundred times during meditation, concentrating fully on its meaning and purpose, so that it will be completely submerged in your subconscious. The word chosen should be positive, such as purity, humility, confidence, courage, love, silence etc.

By repeating certain sentences or a word, a specific command is given to the subconscious in a well-organised manner. In due course, thanks to the tremendous potential of the subconscious, the wishes of the meditator will be translated into reality in a surprising manner.

14. Creative Dynamic Meditation

This meditation blends a variety of meditational techniques. Those who suffer from acute and chronic stress may practise this technique to greater advantage.

This meditation can be practised either in the sitting posture or lying down. If you lie down you may tend to sleep. Those who do not get sleep due to stress and tension may practise this to get peaceful sleep.

It is a **lengthy one**. What you can do is ask one of your friends to read the following text and you may follow his instructions. A better way is to find a person whose voice is good and the whole text may be taped in his voice. During meditation you may listen to the tape and follow the instructions.

Alternatively you may procure the audiotape STRESS MANAGEMENT THROUGH MEDITATION from Tap Foundation International and listen to the tape during meditation. The following is the text of Creative Dynamic Meditation:

Sit comfortably. Close your eyes. Keep all your limbs loose and limp. Don't feel any tension in any part of your body. Don't open your eyes until I ask you to open them.

Now be aware of the sound you are able to hear. (Leave a pause of two minutes to listen to the sound.) This is called Sabdha (sound) Meditation.

Be aware of your thought processes. (Leave a pause of two minutes to be attentive to the thought processes.) This is Chitta Meditation.

Be aware of your breathing processes. (Another two minutes for breathing processes.) This is Vipassana Meditation.

Now be aware of the existence of your entire physical body. Your whole body should be the object of your awareness. Relax your body mentally. Feel the sensation of total relaxation in your whole body – total and complete relaxation.

Again be aware of your breathing process – feel the sensation of breathing through both nostrils.

Feel the coolness of the air that you breathe in – now feel the cool air that you breathe in. Feel the warm air that you breathe out – the air that you breathe out should be warmer. Feel the difference in the temperature of the air that you breathe in and breathe out. The breathe-in air is cool and the breathe-out is warm.

Now mentally imagine that you are breathing in through the left nostril – you are breathing in through the left nostril. Again mentally imagine that you are breathing out through the right nostril.

You are not physically manipulating the nostril breath but using only your imagination. Again breathe in through the right nostril – breathe in through the right nostril – then breathe out through the left nostril, breathe out through the left nostril.

Breathe in through the left nostril – breathe out through the right nostril – breathe in through the right nostril and breathe out through the left nostril – breathe in through the left nostril and breathe out through the right nostril – breathe in through the right nostril and breathe out through the left nostril – this is similar to Nadi Shodhana Pranayama without physically manipulating the nostrils, using only imagination to operate the nostril breath.

This is called psychic breathing. You are mentally manipulating your breathing processes through alternate breathing. This would facilitate your using both sides of the brain. The left side of the brain takes care of the routine way of thinking, analysing and logical reasoning and the right side deals with intuition, creativity and imagination. In order to achieve something great and outstanding in life we should learn to use both sides of the brain. **Psychic breathing** is a marvellous technique to achieve this result. Continue the psychic breathing on your own until I give you further instructions. (Leave a pause of two minutes.)

You are now totally relaxed, completely relaxed, totally relaxed and completely relaxed, your whole body is totally relaxed and completely relaxed.

This is the time for you to repeat your Sankalpa – your resolve to become something great in life – your resolve should be simple and precise – if your objective is to manage stress very effectively, you may resolve to get rid of your stress and attain happiness – for this you may repeat the words BE HAPPY, BE JOLLY, BE CHEERFUL. Repeat this again and again at least five times.

Now again, be aware of your body – your whole body from top to bottom – from head to foot – be aware of your whole body.

Now you are going to enter into another area of consciousness. You rotate your consciousness over different parts of your body.

As I tell you of different parts of the body, you have just to be aware of the physical parts of your body – don't concentrate on any one part of the body – as I proceed, you should also shift your consciousness as fast as possible.

You may mentally name the parts of the body: Be aware of your right hand, right hand thumb, right hand first finger, middle finger, ring finger, little finger. Now be aware of your left hand, left hand thumb, left hand first finger, middle finger, ring finger, little finger.

Now be aware of your head – the hair on your head – your forehead, your right eye, right eyebrow, your left eye, your left eyebrow, your right ear, your left ear, your nose, your right nostril, your left nostril, your mouth, your upper lip, your lower lip, your tongue, your teeth.

Now be aware of your chest, your heart, your lungs, the ribs on your chest, your right shoulder, your right elbow, your left shoulder, your left elbow, your stomach, intestinal organs in your stomach.

Now, be aware of your right leg, left leg, right thigh, left thigh, right calf muscles, left calf muscles, your right sole, your left sole, right toes, left toes.

Now, be aware of your whole body – feel your whole body is very heavy – your whole body is very heavy – feel the heaviness of your whole body.

Be aware of your whole body – your whole body – feel the lightness of your whole body – lightness of your body – your whole body is very light – very light.

Now be aware of your whole body – feel that the body is very cold – feel the chill in your body – feel that the body is very cold – your body is very cold – you feel like shivering – the body is very cold.

Now be aware of your whole body – from top to bottom – feel that the body is very hot now – feel the heat in the body – heat in the body – the whole body is very hot – the body is very hot.

Again be aware of your whole body – from top to bottom – from head to toes – be aware of your whole body – be aware of your whole body.

Now be aware of your breathing process – you are breathing in and breathing out – breathing in and breathing out – be aware of your breathing process.

Now count your breathing cycle –

Breathe in............breathe out............1

Breathe in............breathe out............2

Breathe in............breathe out............3

Breathe in............breathe out............4

Breathe in............breathe out............5

6...7...8...9...10 and then reverse...

10, 9, 8, 7, 6, 5, 4, 3, 2, 1.

Now, be aware of your whole body – your whole body is totally relaxed – completely relaxed – no tension in any part of your body.

The mind is calm and peaceful, tranquil and serene, cool and collected – you have a wonderful feeling all over your body.

With the relaxed frame of mind use your imagination – imagine that you are walking along the road – both sides of the road are full of trees – tall trees – you are walking along the road lined with trees.

Now, you find a beautiful park – a wonderful park which you had not seen so far in your life – the park is filled with fragrant flowers – what an enchanting fragrance of the flowers – you simply enjoy the smell of the flowers – the park is totally empty – no one is there in the park – you are all alone – there is a marble bench in the park – the atmosphere is very calm and quiet – the sky is very clear – there are not many clouds in the sky – you enjoy its journey in the sky – a flock of birds are flying across the sky – everything is peaceful, calm and quiet – it is a wonderful place to meditate.

What a nice place to meditate – mentally repeat the word SOHAM – SOHAM – you synchronise this word with your breathing process.

Breathe in............SO

Breathe out............HAM

Breathe in............SO

Breathe out............HAM

You feel wonderfully relaxed – completely relaxed – you feel the sensation of total relaxation.

Make sure you are not sleeping – you are awake – you are fully conscious – you are not sleeping – you are awake – you are fully conscious.

Now, follow my instructions carefully – I shall be naming a few objects and you should simply recollect those objects – you should bring those objects to your mental consciousness – as I mention the objects you should be able to bring those objects to your mental consciousness.

Table-cycle-book-elephant-lake-boat-paper-aeroplane-mountain-rat-TV-telephone-trees-window-bird-tiger-box-sunrise-bridge-ocean-sand-candle-tomato-tumbler-honey-toilet-train-house-car-shoe-watch-pencil-wastepaper basket-gem clip-calling bell-lorry-computer-flask-wall clock-snow-capped mountain-gold chain-gum bottle-tube light-cow-road-star-palace-village-tray-magnifying glass-hotel-specks-visiting cards-biscuits-rope-soap-temple-punching machine-fan-grapes-bottle-shaving set-jug-mirror-moon-dog-typewriter-currency notes-envelope-cat-church-bureau-curtain-barber shop-swimming pool-cinema theatre-airport-football ground-mosque.

A small girl weeping bitterly – water gushing from a leaked pipe – an old man walking slowly on the road – a car moving at fantastic speed – tennis match in full swing – birds flying across the sky – a beggar eating food with gusto – a woman sitting in a park and discussing things – a small child playing in the middle of the road – a cyclist whistling and riding quite happily – downpour of rain – snow falling – five people climbing a mountain – wall clock ticking five – are you awake – don't sleep – listen to my instructions – now feel the sensation of taking bath – pouring warm water on your body – now wipe away the water after bath – you are now in the warm sun – feel the sensation of travelling in a car – do you hear the sound of a temple bell – you are now writing a letter to your friend – you are posting that letter in the mail box – you are now in a departmental store, buying toothpaste for your use – you are now watching a cricket match on TV.

Be aware that you are sitting in a chair – you are now listening to my instructions – be aware of your breathing – you are breathing in and breathing out – you are now fully relaxed – you are now fully relaxed – relax... relax... relax... Take your hands. Gently rub your eyes.

Slowly open your eyes – calmly and quietly open your eyes...

Significance of this Technique

This is a powerful way to gain total relaxation of both body and mind. The mind is made to switch over from one item to another without allowing it to ponder or reflect over any personal problems, difficulties and sufferings. Stress is nothing but reflecting in our consciousness about personal problems and difficulties, either actual or imagined. People suffering from acute stress may practise this meditation everyday.

15. CRVR Meditation

Dr Carl Simonton of USA has cured several terminal cancer patients by applying the techniques of meditation. His approach is very scientific, logical and effective. Cancer is generally considered incurable. However, he has succeeded in helping many cancer patients who were considered beyond remedy. We shall call his methodology CRVR Meditation: C for Conviction, R for Relaxation, V for Visualisation and R for Radiation.

Conviction: The mind plays a tremendous role in health and disease. People should be convinced of the efficacy of meditation. Therefore, the first step taken by Dr Simonton was to convince his patients that it was possible to cure even terminal cancer through meditation. Before taking up regular treatment, patients were made to believe in their mental power.

Relaxation: Meditational techniques were used to relax patients. Meditation is one of the most powerful ways to relax both body and mind. The patients were made to relax through meditation for a short while. However, this has to be done at frequent intervals. Meditating at frequent intervals facilitates the patients always being in a relaxed mood with alpha waves of the mental state. This is essential for the curative process.

Visualisation: Another powerful facet of the mind is visualisation. What the mind can visualise, the body will literally follow. Visualisation is nothing but imagination with a purpose. When imagination is used to attain an objective it becomes visualisation. Use your imagination to create a mental picture in our mind. When the picture is created without any purpose it becomes daydreaming. If it is done with conscious effort to achieve something it becomes visualisation.

Dr Simonton has used the faculty of visualisation for curing terminal cancer patients. He asked his patients to visualise their cancerous growth and imagine for themselves that the cancerous growth was being reduced day by day, as they use visualisation with tremendous conviction while totally relaxed. They have to do this as frequently as possible everyday. Their mind must be fully saturated with the feeling that their cancer is being cured gradually but definitely.

Radiation: It is very difficult to bring conviction among patients that only through meditation and visualisation a deadly disease like cancer can be cured. Therefore, Dr Simonton ingeniously treated patients with radiation as well. Treating them with the traditional methods encouraged them to believe in his method of treatment. The patients treated with radiation and medication alone did not get cured but patients who practised meditation and visualisation in addition were completely cured. All the patients who had a strong will to survive recovered.

16. Digital Meditation

The purpose of meditation is to shift your consciousness from yourself to something else. A variety of techniques are available in this connection. They are being attentive to sound; chanting mantras; awareness of the breathing cycles; gazing at an object; awareness of one's own thoughts, feelings and actions, etc.

The Digital Meditation that I introduce in this book is unique and very effective. Here one has to register and reproduce 100-digit random numbers as given below:

1	**2**	**3**	**4**	**5**	**6**	**7**	**8**	**9**	**10**
25	01	88	68	14	09	98	60	74	23
11	**12**	**13**	**14**	**15**	**16**	**17**	**18**	**19**	**20**
77	02	18	05	21	04	99	63	67	41
21	**22**	**23**	**24**	**25**	**26**	**27**	**28**	**29**	**30**
75	63	29	10	53	84	29	11	59	31
31	**32**	**33**	**34**	**35**	**36**	**37**	**38**	**39**	**40**
62	05	71	93	28	62	02	31	68	20
41	**42**	**43**	**44**	**45**	**46**	**47**	**48**	**49**	**50**
87	92	20	31	81	76	24	59	12	19

This technique of memorising and reproducing a 100-digit random number is offered in my 30-hour programme 'Creative Memory and Mind Management'. Everyone can register and reproduce a series of numbers. This is possible via another technique called Memory Filing System, which I innovated in the recent past.

The features of this meditation are:

- Write down a series of numbers, preferably a set of one hundred random numbers as shown above.
- Fresh numbers are to be written every time you wish to meditate.
- Read and register the numbers by using the Memory Filing System. Then reproduce the numbers in the same order either silently or by writing on paper.
- The process of registering and reproducing a set of hundred digits may take about 15 minutes for those who have been practising regularly. For beginners it may take more than 30 minutes.
- One can reproduce the numbers in the same order, both forward and backward. The numbers can also be reproduced at random.
- Intense concentration is required.
- It can be considered a **heightened form of meditation**.
- While registering and reproducing the numbers you would be **able to reach alpha waves of mental state**.
- This may be the only meditative technique on this planet that will enable you to **quantitatively measure the qualitative impact of your meditative practice**.

The technique of Memory Filing System is explained in my forthcoming book, *Creative Memory and Mind Management*. Space constraints in this book do not allow me to explain this technique, as an elaborate explanation is required.

A Few Practical Hints

Meditation should be practised as a way of life, rather than a mere ceremony to be performed piously at an appointed time. Efforts should be made to occupy the mind fully with pure and positive thoughts.

Any stressful thoughts and negative feelings that intrude into the mind should be observed in an objective manner like a total stranger. Be aware of your thoughts and feelings all the time in your wakeful state.

Such an awareness alone constitutes a form of meditational technique.

The mind should be allowed to attend to only one thing at a time.

Instead of brooding over personal problems, it is better to concentrate on constructive activities that bring some beneficial results to humanity at large.

The mind should always be saturated with the theme **Love for all and hatred towards none**. No event, howsoever adverse, should disturb the mind, which must always be peaceful, tranquil and serene. This is the state without tension and stress. **A stress-free mind develops your health and personality to a considerable extent.**

OOO

Bibliography

ABHEDANANDA, SWAMY, ***Yoga Psychology*** – Ramakrishna Vedanta Math, 1967

ADIDEVANANDA, ***Yoga as Therapeutic Fact*** – University of Mysore, 1966

ALAIN, ***Yoga for Perfect Health***; Ed. 7 – Pyramid Books

ALEXANDER F.J., ***In the Hours of Meditation*** – Advaita Ashrama, 1973

AMALADAS, BRAHMACHARI, ***Yoga and Contemplation*** – Shantivanam Ashram, 1974

AMALORPAVA Das, D.S., (Ed) – ***Praying Seminar*** – National Biblical Catechetical and Liturgical Centre

ANTHONY ELANJIMATTAM, ***The Yoga Philosophy of Patanjali*** – St. Paul's Publication, 1974

APPAPANT, ***Surya Namaskar*** – Sangam Books, 1970

AUROBINDO, ***Lights on Yoga*** – Aurobindo Ashram, 1974

AUROBINDO, ***Yoga and its Objects*** – Aurobindo Ashram, 1972

ARVIND AND SHANTA, ***Tantra – the Secret Power of Sex*** – Jaico Publishing House, 1976

BAKER M.E. PENNY, ***Meditation – a Step Beyond – Edgar Cayce*** – Pinnacle Books, 1977

BEHANAN, KOVOOR T., ***Yoga: A Scientific Evolution*** – Dover Publication, 1964

BHATT V.M., ***Yogic Powers and God Realisation*** – Bharatiya Vidya Bhavan, 1975

BLOOMFIELD HAROLD & OTHERS, ***TM: Discovering Inner Energy and Overcoming Stress*** – Dell Publishing Co. Inc., 1975

BRUNTON, PAUL, ***Hidden Teachings Beyond Yoga*** – B.I. Publications

BUDHANANDA, SWAMI, ***Mind and Its Control*** – Advaita Ashrama, 1974

CARR, RACHEL E., ***Yoga*** – William Collins and Co. Ltd, 1972

CHAPMAN, A.H. AND OTHERS, ***What TM Can and Cannot do for You*** – Berkley Publishing Corporation, 1976

CHETANAND, YOGI, ***Sex and Yoga*** – Hind Pocket Books, 1977

CHINMAYANANDA, ***Meditation and Life*** – Chinmayananda Publication Trust, 1962

CRISP, TONY, ***Yoga and Childbirth*** – Sphere Books Ltd, 1976

DAY, HARVEY, ***Executive Yoga*** – Pinnacle Books

DAY, HARVEY, ***Practical Yoga*** – Thorsons Publishers, 1968

DAY, HARVEY, ***Yoga Illustrated Dictionary*** – Jaico Publishing House, 1974

DECHANET, ***Christian Yoga*** – Search Press

DECHANET, ***Yoga in Ten Lessons*** – Search Press

DECHANET, ***Yoga and God*** – Search Press

DHIRENDRA BRAHMACHARI, ***Yoga – Yogic Suksma Vyayama*** – Hind Pocket Books, 1975

DIGAMBERJI, SWAMI, ***Collected Papers on Yoga*** – Kaivalyadhama

DONAT, LILIAN K., ***Unisex Yoga*** – Marshall Cavendish Publications, 1976

DUNNE, DESMOND, ***Yoga for Everyone*** – Four Square Books, 1966

DUNNE, DESMOND, ***Yoga Made Easy*** – Prentice Hall, 1974

DUKES, SIR PAUL, ***Yoga of Health, Youth and Joy*** – Haper and Brothers, 1970

ELIZABETH, HAICH, ***Sexual Energy and Yoga*** – George Allen and Unwin, 1972

FEUERSTEIN, G.A., ***Essence of Yoga*** – Rider and Company, 1974

GARDE, R.K., ***Biodynamics of Shadanga Yoga*** – D.B. Taraporavala and Sons

GARDE, R.K., ***Principles and Practice of Yoga Therapy*** – D.B. Taraporavala, 1975

GITANANDA, SWAMY, ***Breath of Life*** – Ananda Ashram

GITANANDA, SWAMY, ***How to Begin Practice of Yoga*** – Ananda Ashram

GITANANDA, SWAMY, ***Intermediate Practices*** – Ananda Ashram

GITANANDA, SWAMY, ***Advanced Yoga Practices*** – Ananda Ashram

GITANANDA, SWAMY, ***Senior Yoga Practices*** – Ananda Ashram

GITANANDA, SWAMY, ***Mudras*** – Ananda Ashram

GITANANDA, SWAMY, ***Yoga Samyama*** – Ananda Ashram

GITANANDA, SWAMY, ***Surya Namaskar*** – Ananda Ashram

GNANESWAR ANAND, ***Yoga for Beginners*** – Sri Ramakrishna Math

GOPI KRISHNA, ***Secret of Yoga*** – Turnstons Books, 1973

GOULD, JOHN, ***Yoga for Health and Beauty*** – Thorsons Publishers, 1972

GOVINDA, LAMA ANAGARIKA, ***Foundations of Tibetan Mysticism*** – B.I. Publications, 1977

GUYOT, FELIX, ***Yoga – the Art and Science of Self-mastery for Success*** – Universal Publications, 1967

HAYDEN, ERIC W., ***Everyday Yoga for Christians*** – Arthur James Ltd

HEWITT JAMES, ***Yoga*** – St. Paul's House

HITTLEMAN, RICHARD L., ***Guide to Yoga Meditation*** – Bantam Books, 1978

HITTLEMAN, RICHARD L., ***Yoga – 8 Steps to Health and Peace*** – Hamlyn Publishing Groups, 1976

HITTLEMAN, RICHARD L., ***Yoga for Physical Fitness*** – Jaico Publications, 1970

HITTLEMAN, RICHARD L., ***Yoga for Personal Living*** – Warner Paperback Library, 1974

HOARE SOPHY, *Yoga* – Macdonald Education Ltd., 1977

HUTCHINSON, RONALD, *Yoga – A Way of Life* – Hamlyn Publishing Group Ltd., 1974

INDIRA DEVI, *Yoga – the Techniques of Health and Happiness* – Jaico Publishing House, 1973

IYENGAR, B.K.S., *Light on Yoga* – George Allen and Unwin, 1974

JOHN MERER, *Asthma and Yoga* – Bihar School of Yoga

JOHN, MUMFORD, *Psychosomatic Yoga* – Aquarian Press, 1974

JOHNSTON, WILLIAM, *Silent Music – the Science of Meditation* – William Collins Sons & Co.

JOSHI, S.K., *Yoga in Daily Life* – Orient Paperbacks, 1976

KENT, HOWARD, *Day-by-Day Yoga* – Hamlyn Publishing Group Ltd., 1974

KRISHNA PREM, SRI, *Initiation into Yoga* – B.I. Publications, 1976

KUVALAYANANDA, SWAMI, *Asanas* – Kaivalyadhama

KUVALAYANANDA, SWAMI, *Pranayama* – Popular Prakashan, 1966

KUVALAYANANDA, SWAMI, *Yogic Therapy* – Government of India, 1971

LYSEBETH, ANDRE V.A., *Yoga – Self-taught* – Vikas Publishing House, 1971

MAHARISHI MAHESH YOGI, *Transcendental Meditation* – Plume Books, 1975

MASCARENHAS B.C.M., *Yoga and Christian Thought* – St. Paul Publications

McCARTNEY, JAMES, *Yoga – the Way of Life* – Rider & Co., 1972

MEENAKSHI DEVI, *Yoga for Expectant Mothers* – Ananda Ashram

MIA, TILLIE, *Get in Touch with Yourself Through Yoga* – Vikas Publishing House, 1974

MONKS OF RAMAKRISHNA ORDER, *Meditation* – Ramakrishna Math, 1975

MURPHET, HOWARD, *Yoga for Busy People* – Orient Longmans, 1971

MUZUMDAR, S., *Yoga Exercises* – Orient Longmans, 1976

NANCY PHELEN & MICHAEL VOLLIN, *Yoga for Women* – Arrow Books, 1972

NORVELL, *Miracle Power of Transcendental Meditation* – D.B. Taraporavala and Sons, 1977

PAVITRA, *On Meditation and Discipline* – Aurobindo Ashram, 1972

PHELAN, NANCY, *Beginners Guide to Yoga* – Sphere Books Ltd., 1976

PHULENDA SINHA, *Yoga – Meaning, Values and Practice* – Jaico Publishing House, 1973

POORNANANDA TIRTHA, SWAMI, *Jnana Sudha* – Jnana Ashram, 1972

POORNANANDA TIRTHA, SWAMI, *Prabodha Sudha* – Jnana Ashram, 1968

PRABHAVANANDA, SWAMI, *Sermon on the Mount According to Vedanta* – Ramakrishna Math, 1972

RAJA RAO, M.R., *Surya Namaskar – Secret of Perfect Health* – Basavagudi, Bangalore, 1960

RAMACHARAKA, *Advanced Course in Yoga Philosophy & Oriental Occultism* – D.B. Taraporavala, 1977

RAMACHARAKA, *Hatha Yoga or Yogic Philosophy of Physical Well-being* – D.B. Taraporavala, 1972

RAMACHARAKA, *Science of Breath* – D.B. Taraporavala, 1974

RELE V.G., *Yogic Asanas for Health and Vigour* – D.B. Taraporavala, 1972

RICHMOND, SONYA, *Commonsense About Yoga* – MacGibbon & Kee Ltd., 1971

RICHMOND, SONYA, *How to be Healthy with Yoga* – Arco Publishing Co. Ltd., 1972

RICHMOND, SONYA, *Yoga and Your Health* – Mayflower Books, 1973

ROSS KAREN, *New Manual of Yoga* – W. Foulsham & Co. Ltd., 1973

SARASWATHI, SWAMY SATYANANDA, *Dynamics of Yoga* – Bihar School of Yoga, 1976

SARASWATHI, SWAMY SATYANANDA, *Asana – Pranayama – Mudra – Bandha* – Bihar School of Yoga, 1973

SARASWATHI, SWAMY SATYANANDA, *Meditation from the Tantra* – Bihar School of Yoga, 1977

SARASWATHI, SWAMY SATYANANDA, *Yoga: From Shore to Shore* – Bihar School of Yoga, 1975

SARASWATHI, SWAMY SANKAR DEVANANDA, *Yogic Management of Asthma, Blood Pressure, Diabetes* – Bihar School of Yoga, 1977

SHARMA, PANDIT SHIV, *Yoga Against Spinal Pain* – B.I. Publications

SHARMA, PANDIT SHIV, *Yoga And Sex* – B.I. Publications, 1973

SHAMBUNATH, PANDIT, *Yoga – A Guide for All* – IBH Publishing Co., 1975

SIDDESHWARANANDA, SWAMI, *Meditation According to Vedanta* – Trichur, 1973

SINGH, S.K., *Life Style – Psychodynamics of Yoga* – Research Institute of Values and Yoga, 1972

SITADEVI, YOGENDRA, *Yoga Simplified for Women* – Yoga Institute, 1972

SIVANANDA, SWAMI, *Concentration and Meditation* – The Divine Life Society, 1975

SIVANANDA, SWAMI, *Practice of Yoga* – The Divine Life Society, 1970

SIVANANDA, SWAMI, *Yoga Asanas* – The Divine Life Society, 1972

SIVANANDA, SWAMI, *Yogic Home Exercises* – D.B. Taraporavala, 1971

SUBHA NARAYANA, *Fundamentals of Yoga* Dipti Publications, 1974

TAIMINI, I.K., *Glimpses into the Psychology of Yoga* – Madras Theosophical Publishing House, 1973

TAIMINI, I.K., *Science of Yoga* – Theosophical Society, 1968

UMESH CHANDRAJI, *Umesh Yoga Dharshan* – Shri Ramathirth Ashram, 1975

VARADACHARI VENKEEPURAM, *Hindu Yoga – Parapsychology and Modern Thought* – Higginbothams (P) Ltd., 1967

VIVEKANANDA, SWAMI, ***Bhakti Yoga*** – Advaita Ashrama, 1970

VIVEKANANDA, SWAMI, ***Karma Yoga*** – Advaita Ashrama, 1970

VIVEKANANDA, SWAMI, ***Jnana Yoga*** – Advaita Ashrama, 1972

VIVEKANANDA, SWAMI, ***Raja Yoga*** – Advaita Ashrama, 1972

VITALDAS, YOGI, ***The Yoga System of Health and Relief from Pain*** – Cornerstone Library, 1973

VISHNUDEVANANDA, SWAMI, ***Complete Illustrated Book of Yoga*** – Pocket Books, 1974

VOLIN MICHAEL & PHELAN NANCY, ***Yoga for Beauty*** – ARC Books Inc., 1971

WOOD, EARNEST, ***Great Systems of Yoga*** – D.B. Taraporavala

WOOD, EARNEST, ***Yoga*** – Penguin Books, 1973

WOODROFFE, SIR JOHN, ***Garland of Letters: Studies in Mantra Sastra*** – Ganesh and Co., 1973

WOODROFFE, SIR JOHN, ***Introduction to Tantra Sastra*** – Ganesh & Co., 1974

WOODROFFE, SIR JOHN – ***Serpent Power,*** Ganesh & Co., 1974

YESUDIEN SELVARAJ & ELIZABETH HAICH, ***Yoga and Health*** – Unwin Books, 1972

YOGACHARYA SHANTIKUMAR, ***The Science of Yogic Breathing*** – Jaico Publishing House, 1974

YOGANANDA, SRI PARAMAHAMSA, ***Autobiography of a Yogi*** – Jaico Publishing House, 1975

YOGENDRA JAYADEVA, ***Yoga Today*** – Macmillan & Co., 1971

YOGENDRA, SRI, ***Facts about Yoga*** – Yoga Institute, 1971

YOGENDRA, SRI, ***Why Yoga*** – Yoga Institute, 1976

YOGENDRA, SRI, ***Yoga Asanas Simplified*** – Yoga Institute, 1973

YOGENDRA, SRI, ***Yoga Essays*** – Yoga Institute, 1959

YOGENDRA, SRI, ***Hatha Yoga Simplified*** – Yoga Institute, 1970

Index

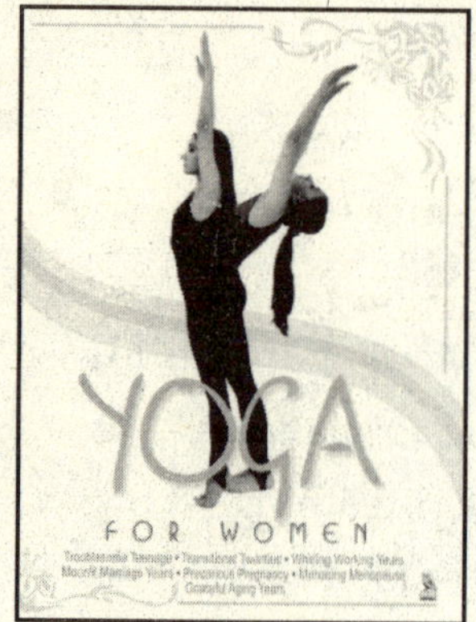

Yoga For Women

—Meghna Virk Bains

There is a famous saying in the Zen religion that 'no teaching worth a name can give the key through words'. It stands true in the case of yoga, where the whole essence lies in its physical and practical experience. However, I believe that words are the verbal embodiment of power. Herein lies my aim of writing this book to reach out to as many wonderful women out there as possible.

Yoga has brought many phenomenal transformations in my life as a woman. I wish to share this blissful journey with you, hoping to help you rediscover your lost potentials and in the process re-establish the connection with the real you.

This might not be the ultimate piece of work on yoga. Nevertheless, I can assure you that in its ordinary nature of description, you might stumble upon the most extraordinary answers. My earnest request to you is to drop all your pre-conceived notions and apprehensions before you embark upon this journey. Remember, it is never too late to learn how to live as long as you are alive.

Pages: 104 • Price: Rs. 150/- • ***Postage: 15/-***

YOGA for HEALTH & PERSONALITY

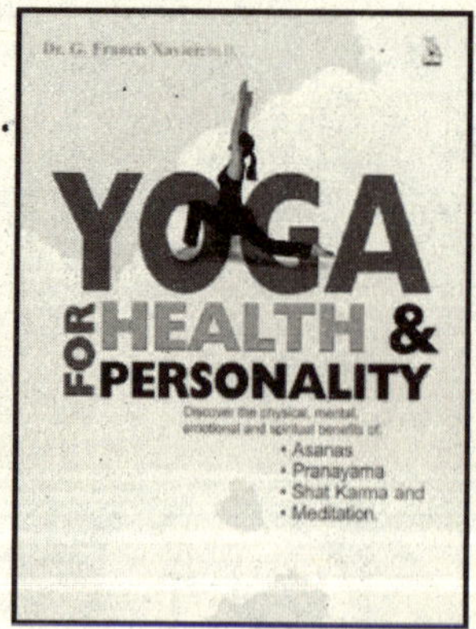

—Dr G. Francis Xavier, Ph.D

Yoga is a holistic science promoting specific techniques for integrated development of man's entire being — physical, mental, emotional and spiritual. Regular practice of yoga ensures sound health, sharp intellect, youthful looks, abundant energy, emotional maturity, composure, compassion and spiritual awareness.

This book is an unmatched work that explores all practical aspects of yoga — Asanas, Pranayama, Shat Karma and meditation. The pages are profusely illustrated with photos of yogic asanas performed by the author and others, making them easy to follow. The step-by-step guidelines explaining the techniques for every posture. The specific benefits of each asana are also stated. Suitable for young and old alike, just half an hour of daily yoga will help you overcome bad habits, improve your personality and make you a better human being in every respect.

Big Size • Pages: 124 • Price: Postage: Rs. 15/-

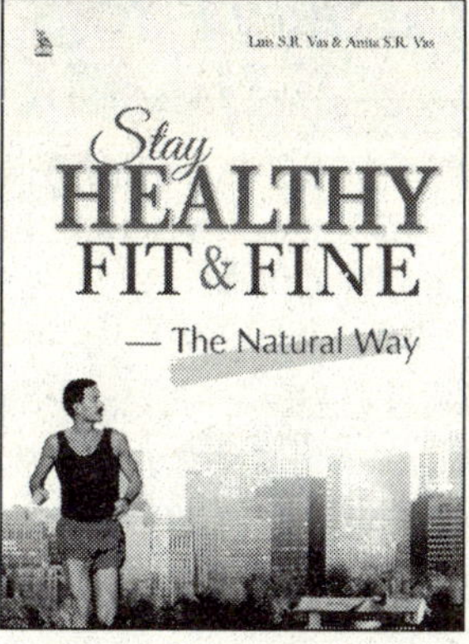

Stay Healthy Fit & Fine

—Luis S.R. Vas & Anita S.R. Vas

Stay Healthy Fit & Fine incorporates research findings on health, psychology, body care and spirituality which emphasise the benefits of natural living. A common theme runs through all the material gathered here. The more you rely on nature and nature therapy in dealing with your physical and mental problems, the more joy you get out of life.

The authors hope the reader will be able to regain natural joy by experimenting with some of the advice from experts presented here which include:

- Coping with stress through relaxation techniques and pleasant and positive thoughts.
- Role of diet in achieving mental & physical well being.
- Safe & successful physical activity program.
- Natural grooming and herbal preparation to attain increased self-confidence.

Pages: 152 • Price: Rs. 120/- • Postage: 15/-

Meditation

The gateway to enhance your health, mental abilities as well as emotional & spiritual well being

—Luis S.R. Vas

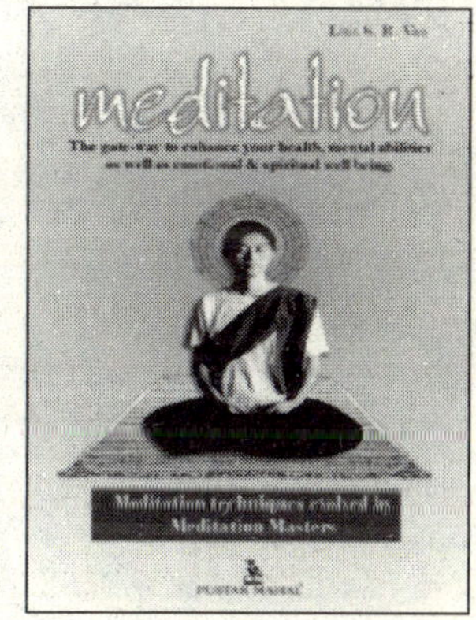

Meditation techniques evolved by Meditation Masters

Meditation is an ancient religious practice, being routinely prescribed in the modern secular society, not just by spiritual masters, but by behavioural scientists, medical practitioners and business consultants. It has found widely varied applications in religious institutions, medical facilities, educational establishments and business organisations. This is a relatively recent development. Less than half a century ago the word meditation, in the sense it is used today, was largely unfamiliar to those outside the Hindu and Buddhist religious traditions.

This book traces the growth of meditation around the world and focuses on several prominent meditation masters who have adapted ancient meditation practices for modern times or developed their own approaches to meditation to enhance health and mental capabilities, as well as emotional and spiritual well-being.

It concludes with a discussion on the benefits of meditation for modern men and women. The reader can try out the various techniques described and decide on the one most suited to his or her own needs.

Pages: 224 • Price: Rs. 96/- • Postage: 15/-

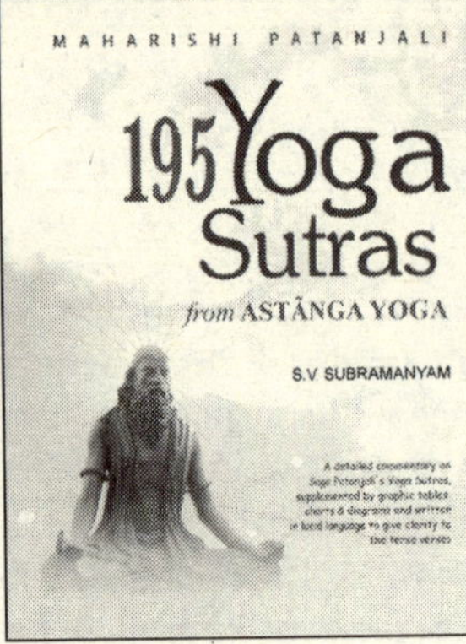

195 Yoga Sutras From Astanga Yoga

—Prof. S. V. Subramanyam

Presents all the 195 Yoga Sutras professed by the legendary Maharishi PATANJALI. He affirmed that Yoga is not only limited to Asanas, but also aims at outer and inner purification; control and balance of the self; meditation and complete absorption. And finally union with the Self.

Contains 4 Chapters: Samadhi; Sadhana; Vibhuti and Kaivalya. Comprises of all the 8 limbs of Ashtanga Yoga: 5 external and 3 internal, Yama; Niyama; Asana; Pranayama; Pratyahara; Dharana; Dhyana; and Samadhi. The book fully utilizes available technology to aid elaboration of the commentary on Yoga Sutras which are admittedly terse.

Charts and tables as well as graphs and pictures adore the book practically on every page so that the reader finds it helpful to enhance his understanding. Stories and quotations from the spiritual greats are added to widen comprehension. This then is a book that is truly unique in its presentation that would find ready acceptance by Yoga teachers and students alike all over the world. All those students and teachers of Yogasanas who wish to go beyond Asanas and aim at avoidance of mental modifications and the resultant stressful life would find this book a boon.

Pages: 364 • Price : Rs. 250/- • Postage: 15/-

WHAT YOU EAT TODAY

—Dr. M. TED MORTER, JR., M.A.

A book that answers all your health problems and ensures a disease-free life WELLNESS • DISEASE PREVENTION • NUTRITION

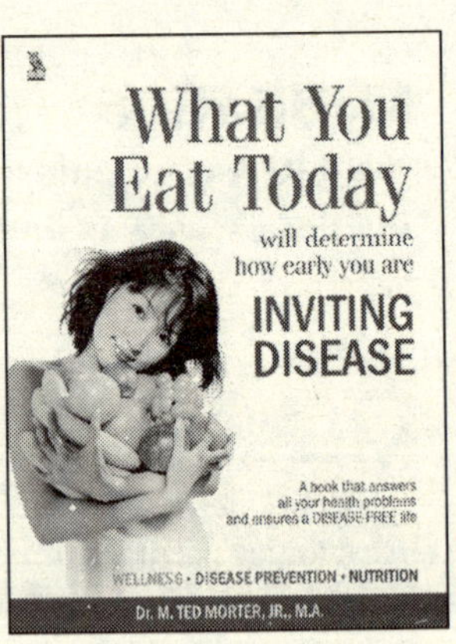

Imagine going through your day without feeling sick or tired. Through this new edition of the bestseller Your Health, Your Choice, you will learn to control how you feel both physically and emotionally. Inside the pages of this revolutionary guide you will discover nutrition guidelines and wellness principles that will help ensure good health and transform the way you feel.

Inside these pages you will discover that:

- The food you ate in the past determines how healthy you will be in the future.
- Age is no excuse for disease, aches or pains.
- You can evaluate your health before symptoms of disease appear.
- Too much protein is hazardous to your health.
- Healing is automatic if you give your body a chance.

Pages: 304 • Price: Rs. 225/- • Postage: 15/-

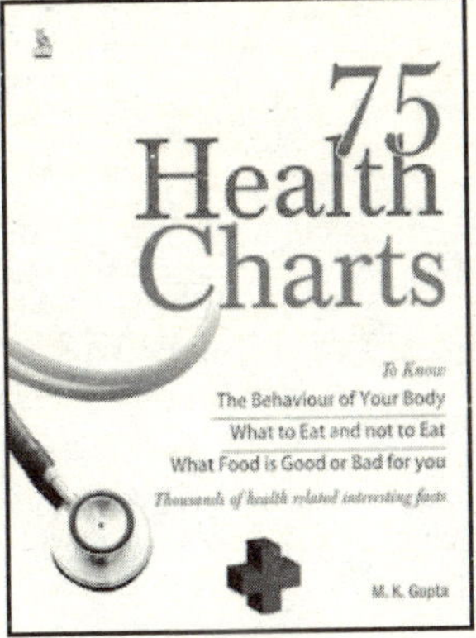

75 HEALTH CHARTS

—M.K. Gupta

As any health-conscious person knows, health is truly wealth. Yet, simply harbouring good intentions does not ensure good health for anyone. Beginning in infancy and right up to our twilight years, a conscious attempt has to be made to lead a healthy lifestyle. In the formative years, our parents make this effort on our behalf. But as we enter the teens and take control of our own destinies, how well informed we are on health-related issues makes all the difference between physical well-being and ill health.

This book ensures you have all the facts, figures and data at your fingertips to promote proper health and nutrition in order to prevent disease. Indeed, the cost of prevention is a pittance compared to the cost of a cure. Towards this end, *75 Health Charts* has it all: height and weight charts, blood pressure and pulse rate charts, calorie charts, fat and cholesterol charts, vitamin and mineral charts, balanced diet charts, pollution health hazard charts, infectious diseases and immunisation charts, healthy heart and stress charts... not to mention other relevant charts, tables and data.

So, if health has always been your problem, this book is just what the doctor ordered. And if health has been your forte, this book is exactly what the doctor would recommend to maintain you in the pink of your health. Either way, *75 Health Charts* is a must-read for all people.

Big Size • Pages: 144 • Price : Rs. 150/- • Postage: Rs. 15/-

YOGA for HEALTH

—N.S. Ravishankar

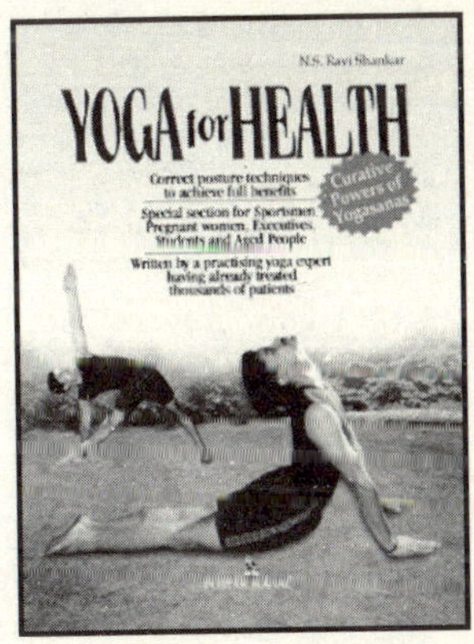

Yoga today is universally acknowledged as a natural way to sound health and overall physical and mental well-being. And given its popularity, a variety of self-help yoga guides are available to the reader. But what makes this book unique is its approach and presentation. The book packs over 100 yogic asanas thoroughly illustrated, and backed by well-designed techniques to perform specific exercises from the first step to the last with each explanation supplemented by the therapeutic advantages of that posture. From how Tadasana gives strength to legs and feet and stimulates nervous system, Garudasana removes cramps in calf muscles, Natarajasana helps to reduce fat, it goes on to explain the benefits of Ardha Chandrasana in strengthening digestive system, and of Vatayanasana in curing joint pain, to list a few.

In addition, the book offers an overview of this age-old science, besides a detailed index of different ailments and the names of asanas useful in curing them. A special chapter is also devoted to specific yogic exercises for Farmers, Pregnant women, Aged people, Artists and Craftsmen, Models, Students, Executives and Sportsmen.

Big Size • Pages: 184 • Price : Rs. 195/- • Postage: Rs. 15/-

CATALOGUE 2016

PUSTAK MAHAL®

J-3/16, Daryaganj, New Delhi-110002
Ph.: 23276539, 23272783-84, Fax: 011-23260518

FREE Tutorial CD

Available in Marathi, Tamil, Telugu, Punjabi also.

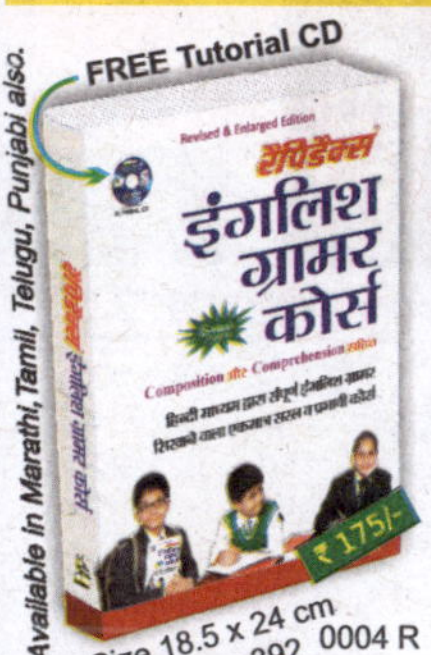

Big Size 18.5 x 24 cm
Pages over 392 0004 R

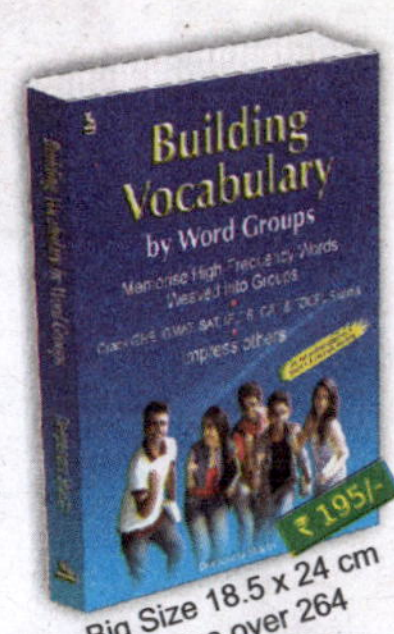

Big Size 18.5 x 24 cm
Pages over 264
8722 F

FREE Tutorial CD

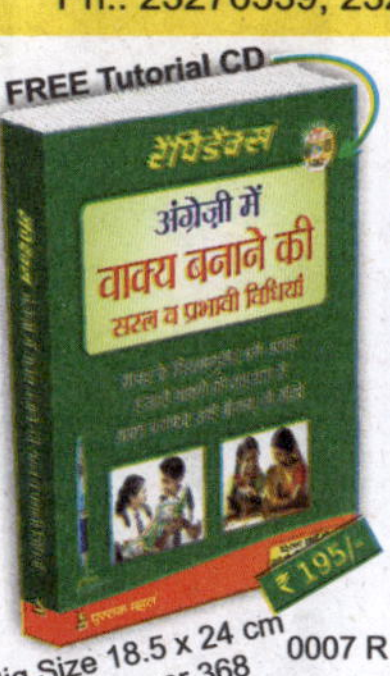

Big Size 18.5 x 24 cm
Pages over 368 0007 R

FREE Tutorial DVD

Available in Tamil, Telugu also

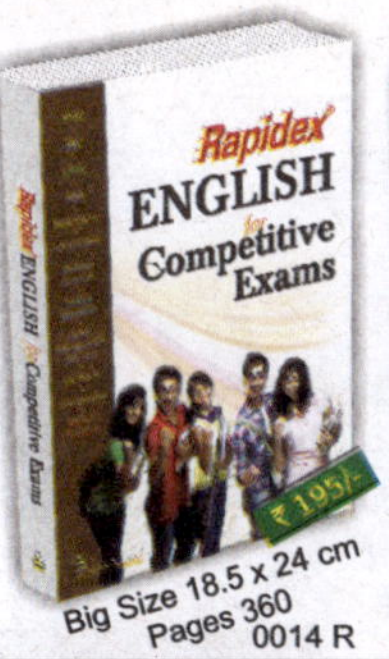

Big Size 18.5 x 24 cm
Pages 384 0001 R

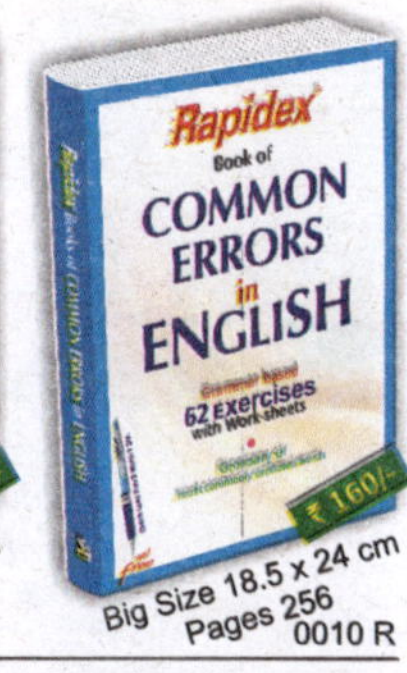

Big Size 18.5 x 24 cm
Pages 360
0014 R

Big Size 18.5 x 24 cm
Pages 256
0010 R

FREE Tutorial CD

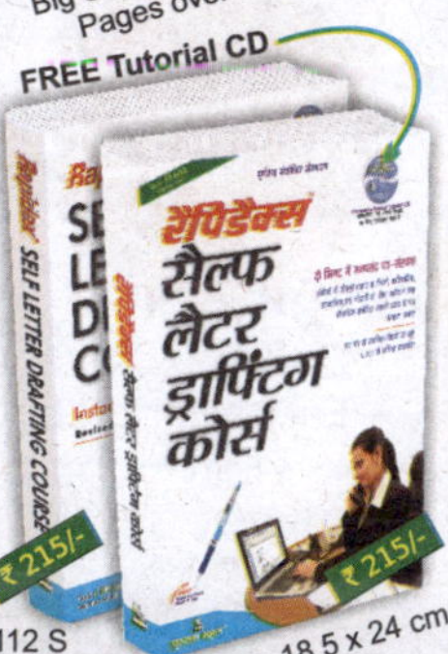

1112 S
0008 R Big Size 18.5 x 24 cm
Pages 388

FREE Tutorial DVD

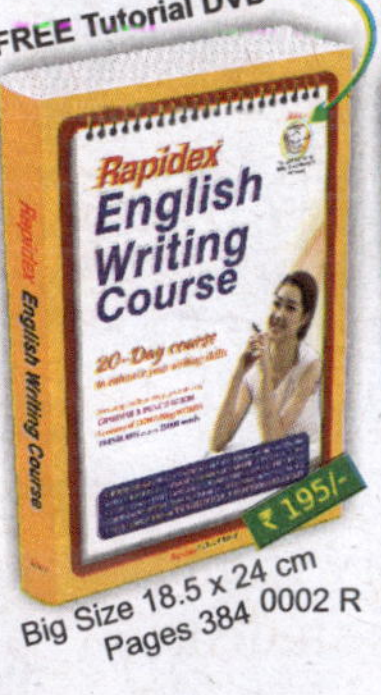

Big Size 18.5 x 24 cm
Pages 384 0002 R

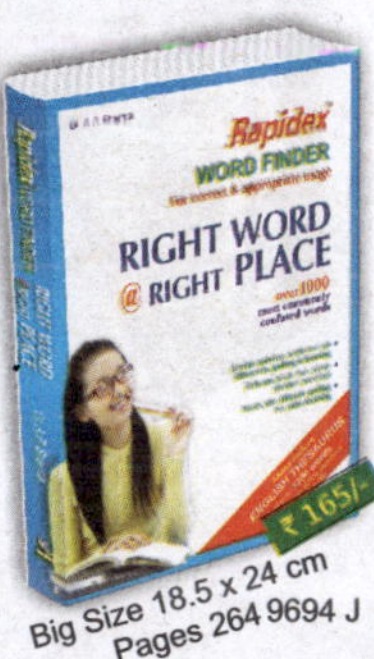

Big Size 18.5 x 24 cm
Pages 264 9694 J

FREE Tutorial CD

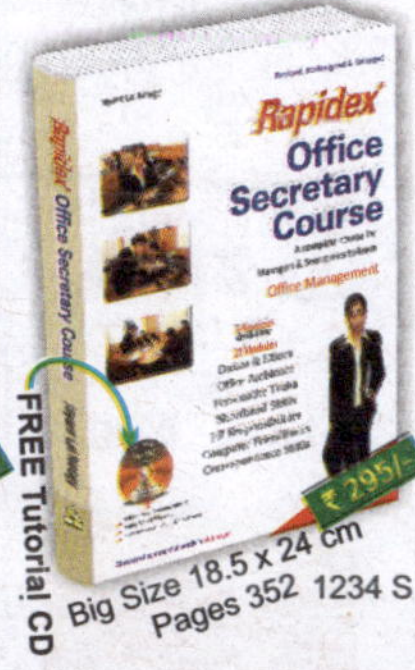

Big Size 18.5 x 24 cm
Pages 352 1234 S

With a CD for learning correct pronounciation of English and other language

Big Size 250 Pages & above in each

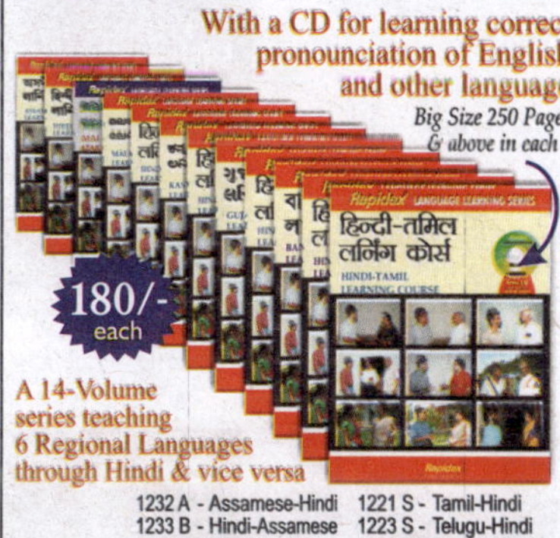

A 14-Volume series teaching 6 Regional Languages through Hindi & vice versa

1232 A - Assamese-Hindi	1221 S - Tamil-Hindi
1233 B - Hindi-Assamese	1223 S - Telugu-Hindi
1215 S - Hindi-Tamil	1224 S - Bangla-Hindi
1217 S - Hindi-Telugu	1225 S - Gujarati-Hindi
1218 S - Hindi-Bangla	1222 S - Kannada-Hindi
1219 S - Hindi-Gujarati	1128 B - Hindi-Arabic
1216 S - Hindi Kannada	1220 S - Malayalam-Hindi
1236 A - Malayalam-Arabic	1214 S - Hindi-Malayalam

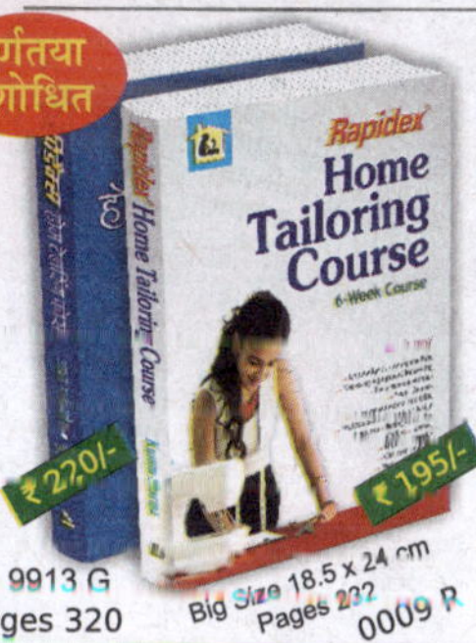

9913 G
Pages 320 Big Size 18.5 x 24 cm
Pages 232 0009 R

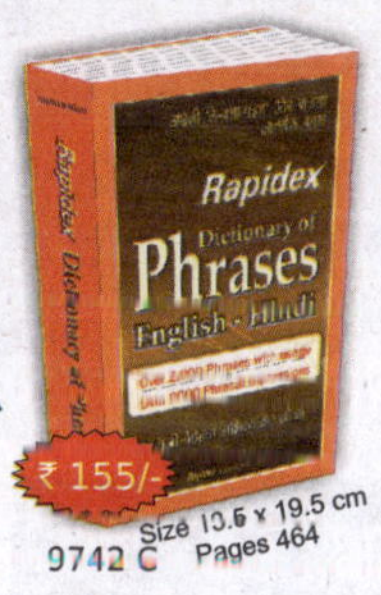

9742 C Size 13.5 x 19.5 cm
Pages 464

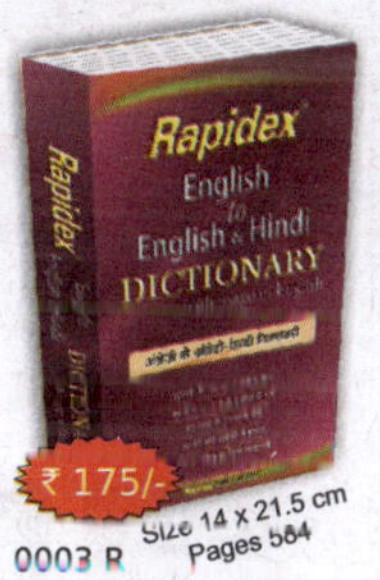

0003 R Size 14 x 21.5 cm
Pages 584

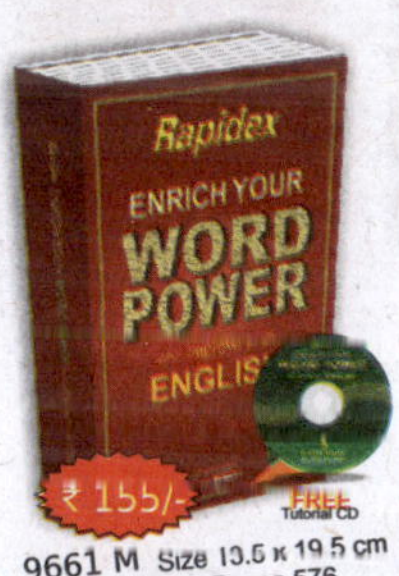

9661 M Size 13.5 x 19.5 cm
Pages 576

Pages 252-256 in each

6611 G - English – Hindi
1131 A - English – Bangla
1132 D - English – Tamil
1134 B - English – Kannada
1136 D - English – Telugu
1137 A - English – Gujarati
1135 C - English – Malayalam

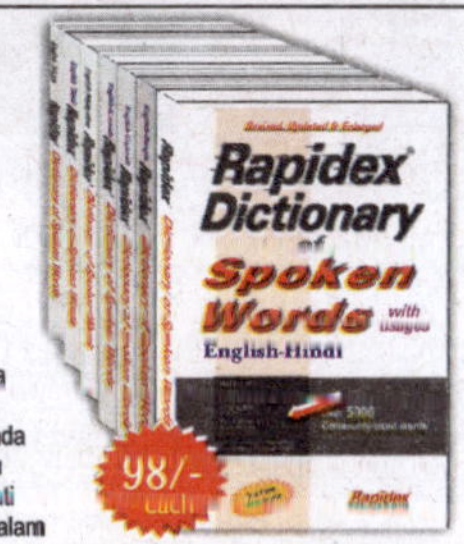

English-Hindi, English-Tamil, English-Kannada
English-Telugu, English-Urdu, English-Assamese
English-Bangla, English-Odia, English-Malayalam
English-Marathi, English-Gujarati

Over 1200 entries with coloured pictures

English-Hindi, English- Marathi
English-Odia, English-Kannada
English-Tamil, English-Telugu
English-Nepali, English Assamese
English-Bangla

अंग्रेज़ी के 10000 से अधिक शब्द
एक शब्द के अनेक अर्थ
अर्थानुसार प्रयोग

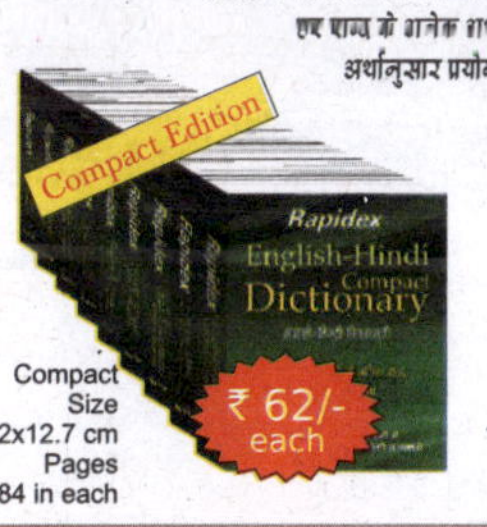

Compact Size 10.2x12.7 cm
Pages 384 in each

English-Hindi, English-Marathi,
English-Odia, English-Kannada,
English-Tamil, English-Telugu,
English-Nepali, English-Bangla
English to Punjabi & Hindi,
English-Assamese

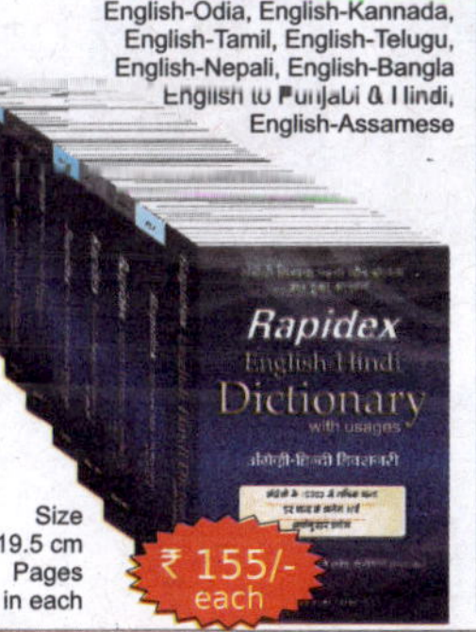

Size 13.5x19.5 cm
Pages 576 in each

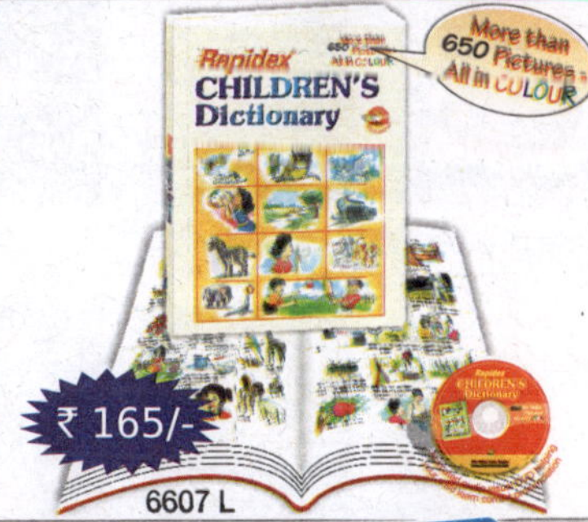

6607 L

Buy online at our website or at Leading Bookshops from:

PUSTAK MAHAL®
Delhi • Mumbai • Patna • Bengaluru
J-3/16, Daryaganj (Opposite Happy School), New Delhi -110002
Fax: 23260510 email: info@pustakmahal.com Website: www.pustakmahal.com

Buy from online Shopping Portals paying CASH ON DELIVERY at your doorstep
flipkart HOMESHOP 18 snapdeal amazon.in uRead.com

Authors/Writers are invited to submit their manuscripts through our website.

POPULAR SCIENCE

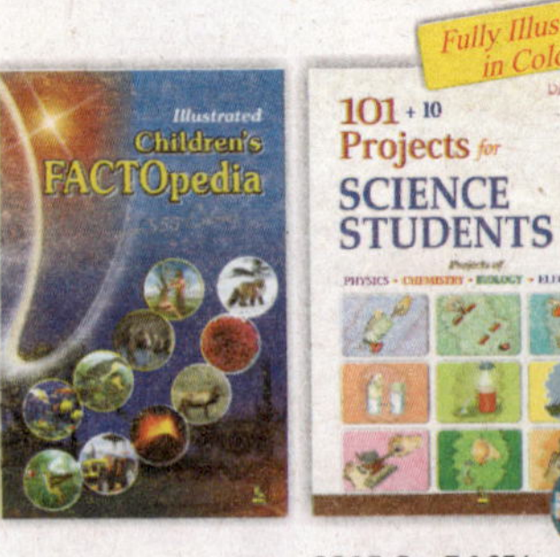

9496 A • Rs. 120/-

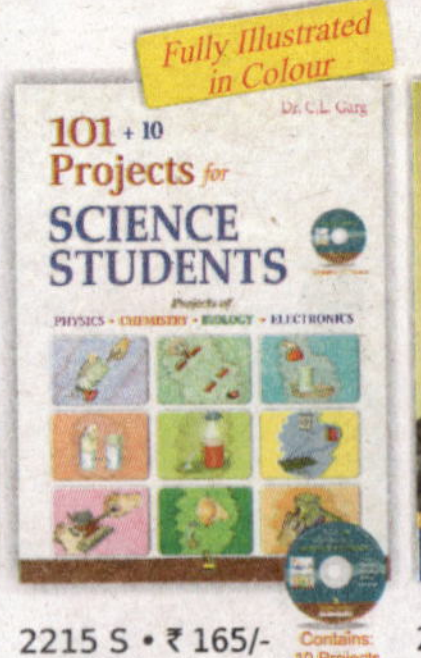

2215 S • ₹ 165/- Available in Hindi also.

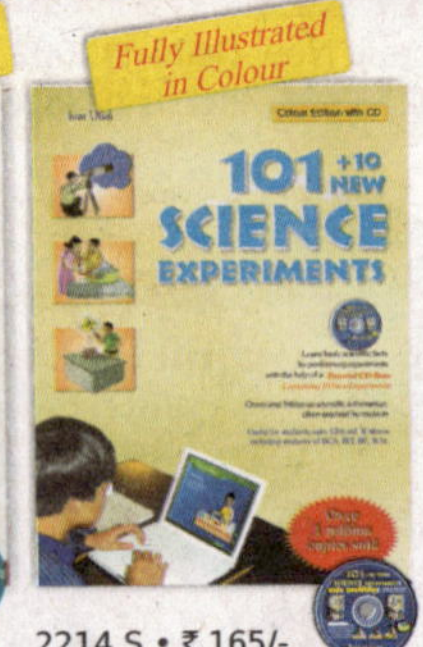

2214 S • ₹ 165/- Available in Hindi also.

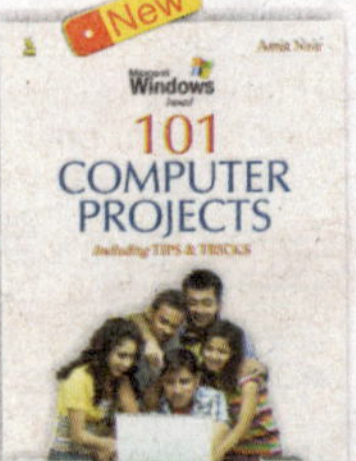

8716 T • ₹ 160/-

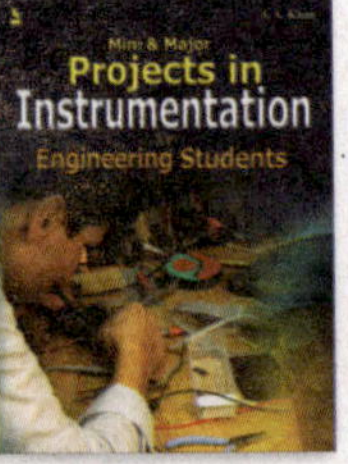

8733 D • ₹ 195/-

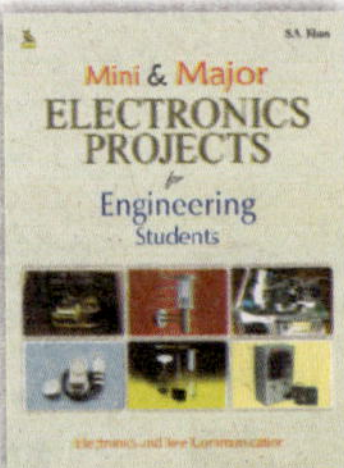

9660 K • ₹ 295/-

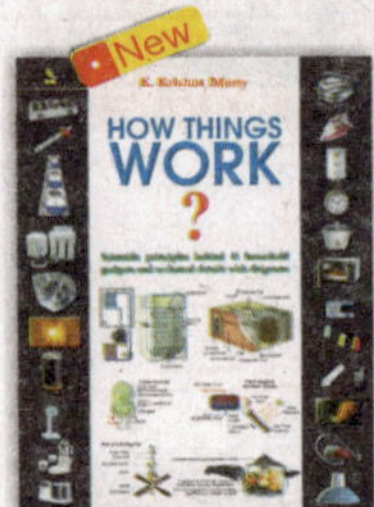

8702 B• ₹ 150/-

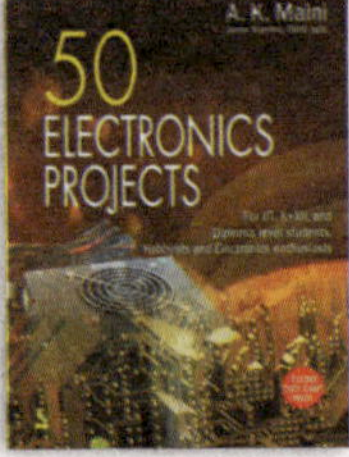

6678 D • ₹ 195/-

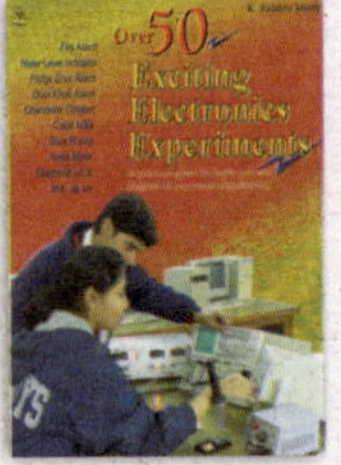

6679 A • ₹ 150/-

QUIZ BOOKS

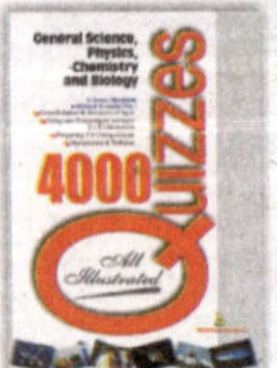

8965 D • ₹ 150/-

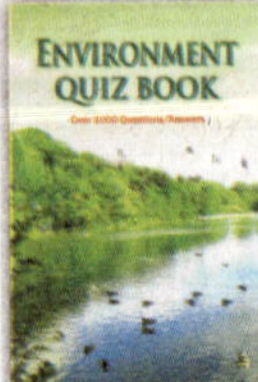

7726 K • ₹ 120/-

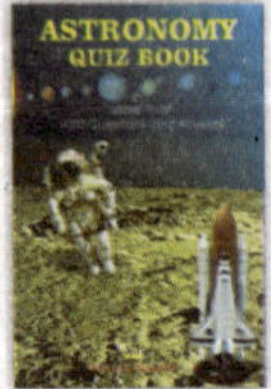

7727 L • ₹ 120/-

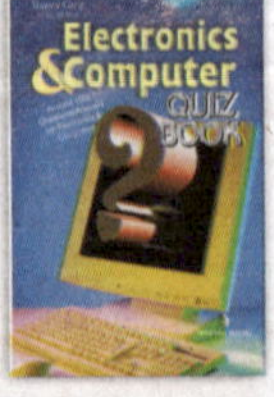

7723 F • ₹ 100/-

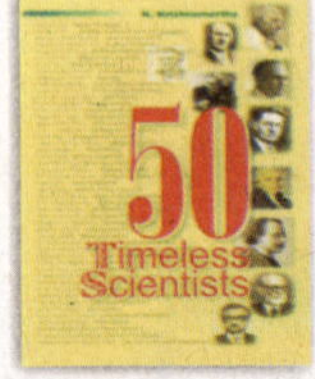

9412 C • ₹ 150/-

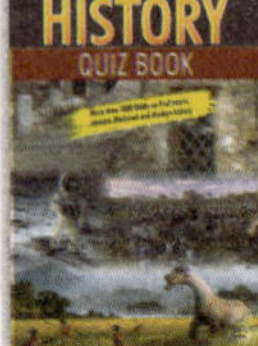

7753 G • ₹ 120/-

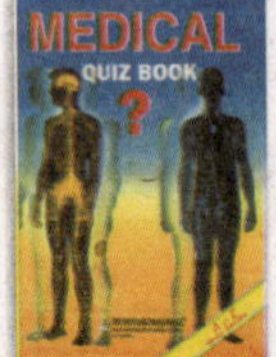

7725 B • ₹ 100/-

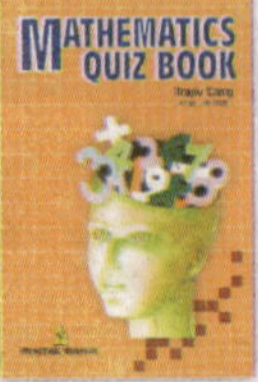

7722 E • ₹ 120/-

NEW RELEASES

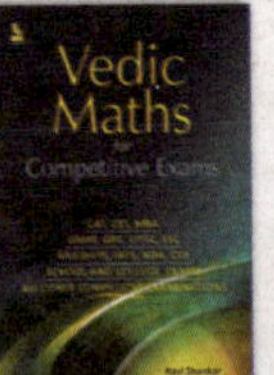

8767 C • Rs. 120/-

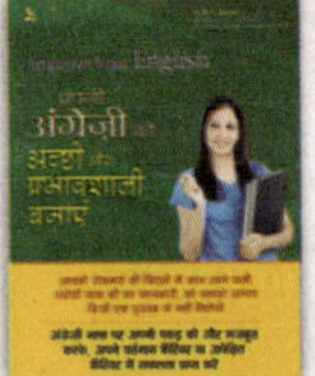

0019 R • Rs. 160/-

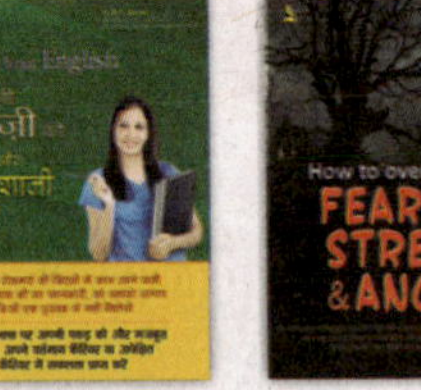

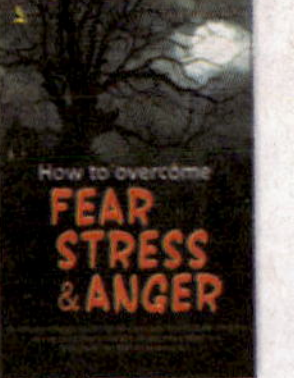

8762 P • Rs. 140/-

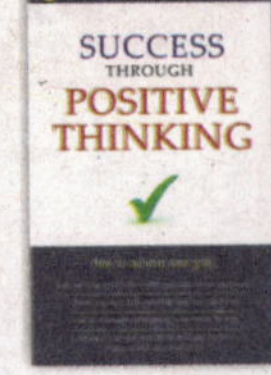

8764 T • Rs. 160/-

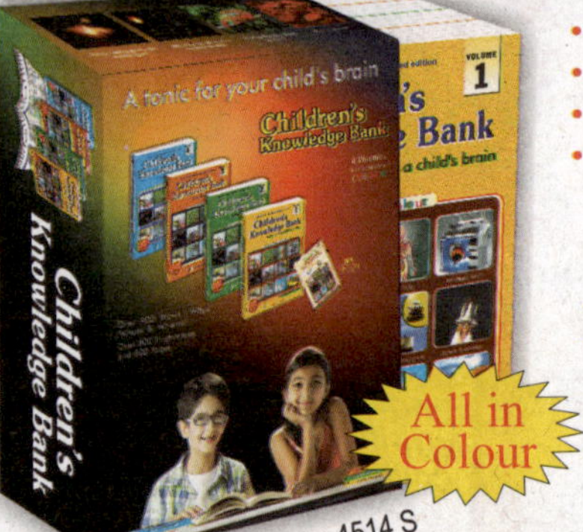

Set Code: 4514 S

- Over 900 Illustrations
- Over 800 Pages
- 890 Articles
- Four Volumes

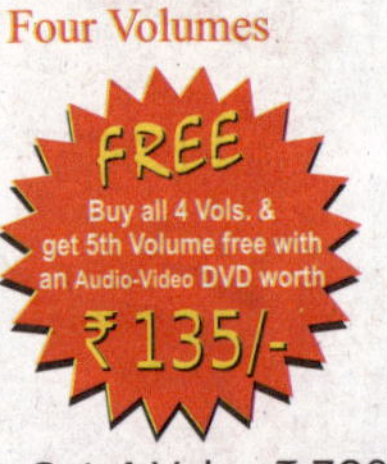

Set 4 Vols.: ₹ 780/-
Each Vol.: ₹ 195/-

Available in Hindi & English both

This Library is must for every student *of a* School *or* *a* College

Also equally useful for everyone else

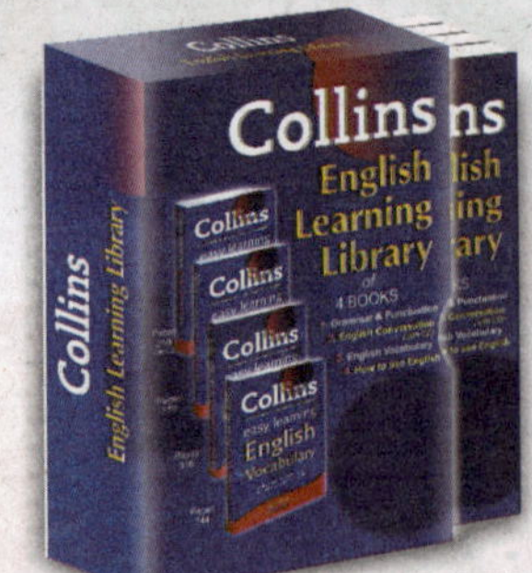

Price: ₹ 600/-

Contains 4 books of ₹ 150/- each

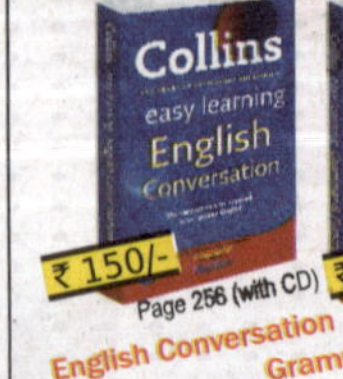

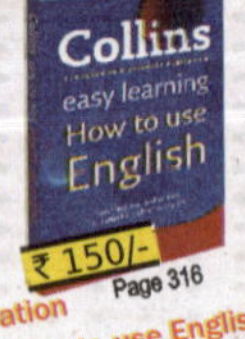

₹ 150/- Page 256 (with CD) English Conversation
₹ 150/- Page 310 Grammar & Punctuation
₹ 150/- Page 316 How to use English
₹ 150/- Page 344 English Vocabulary

4 Books of the Library

Miscellaneous

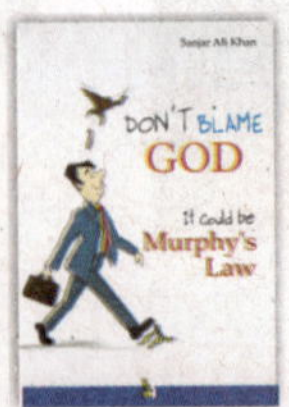

9497 B • ₹ 120/-

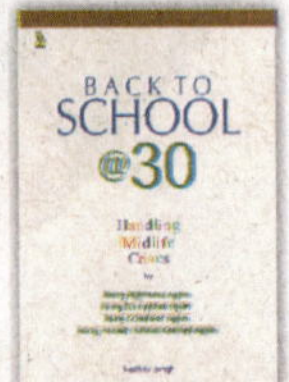

9783 H • ₹ 150/-

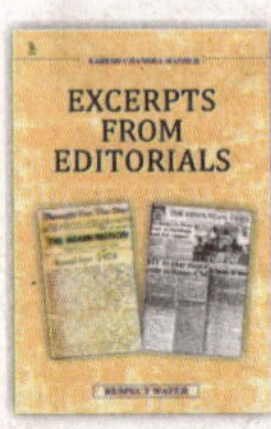

9680 B • ₹ 295/-

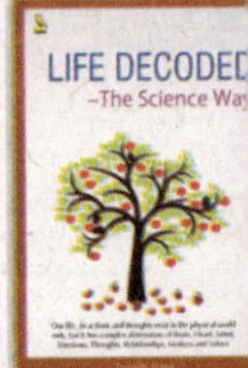

9686 H • ₹ 120

SELF-IMPROVEMENT

New

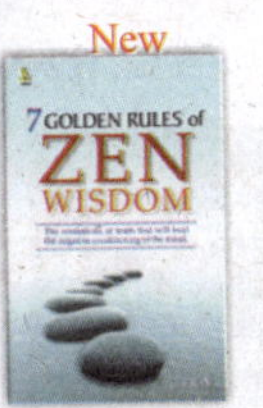

9698 R • ₹ 195/-

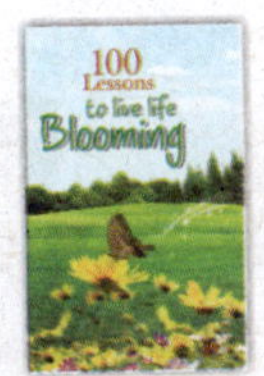

9498 C • ₹ 180/-

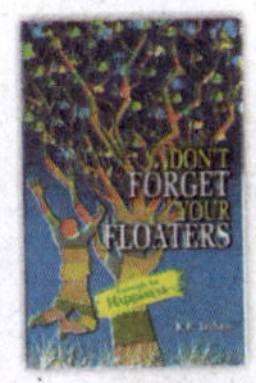

9490 H • ₹ 175/-

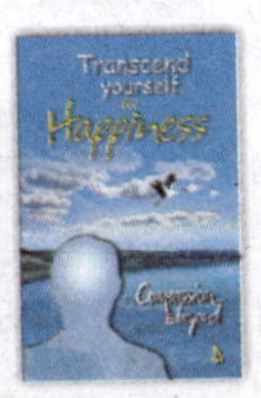

9464 R • ₹ 80/-

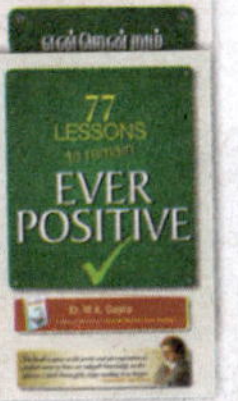

9096 B • ₹ 150/-

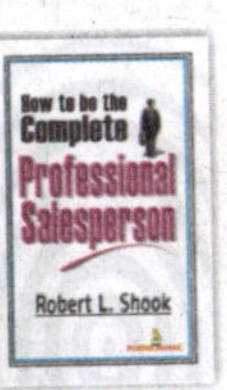

5614 E • ₹ 150/-

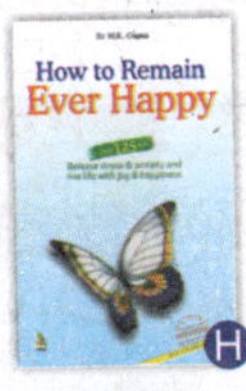

4008 J • ₹ 150/-

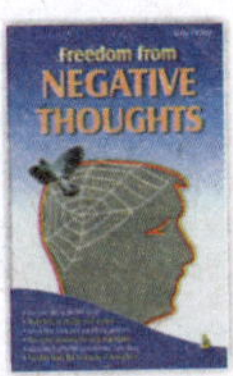

9026 D • ₹ 120/-

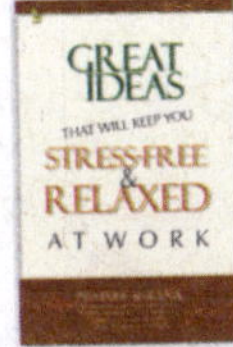

9786 M • ₹ 195/-

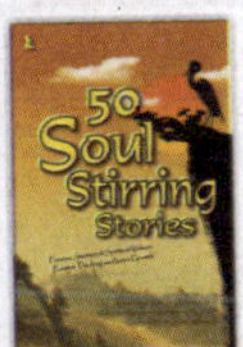

9491 J • ₹ 100/-

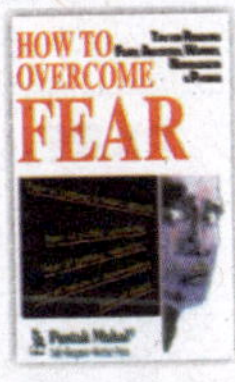

8885 D • ₹ 150/-

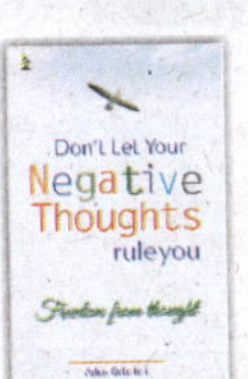

9081 D • ₹ 150/-

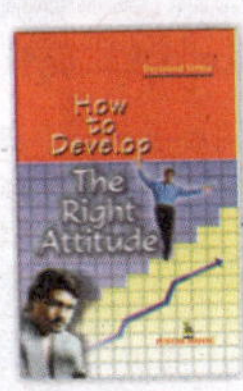

9091 B • ₹ 120/-

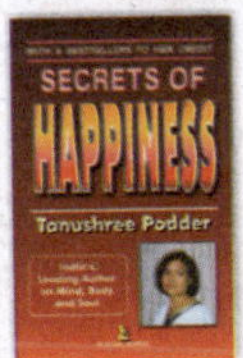

9060 B • ₹ 195/-

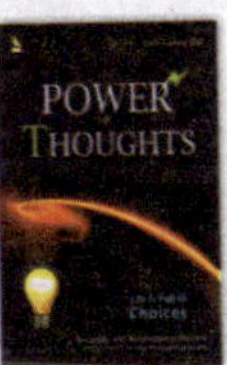

9684 F • ₹ 195/-

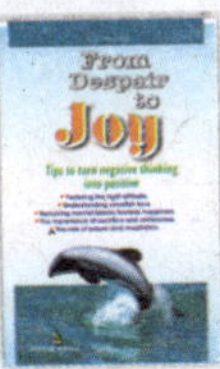

8928 D • ₹ 80/-

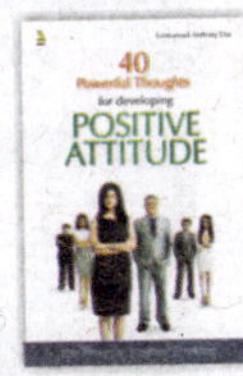

9449 A • ₹ 195/-

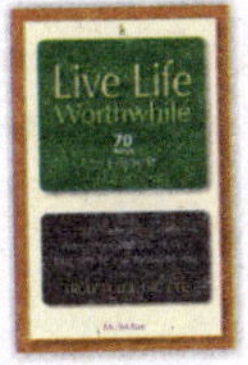

9788 R • ₹ 195/-

MANAGEMENT/JOB/CARRIER/BUSINESS & PROFESSION

All Time Bestsellers

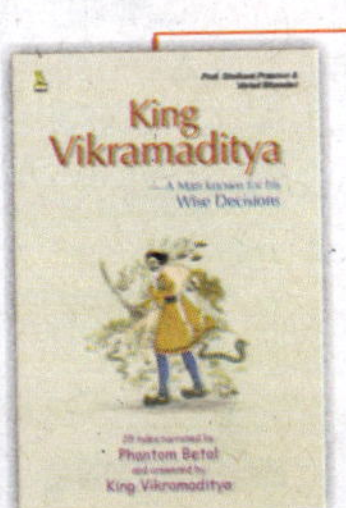

9461 K • ₹ 150/-

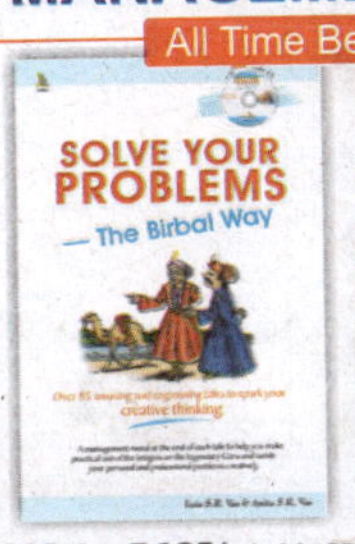

5338 A • ₹ 135/- (with CD)

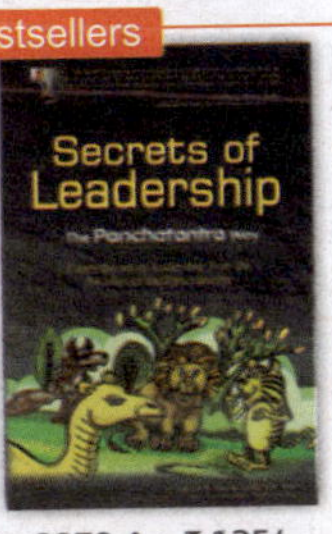

8979 A • ₹ 135/-

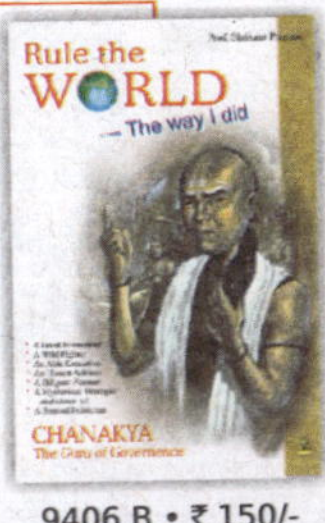

9406 B • ₹ 150/-

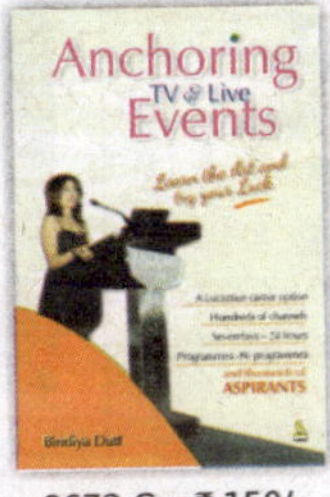

9672 G • ₹ 150/-

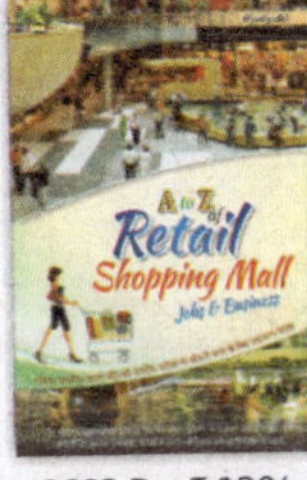

9682 D • ₹ 120/-

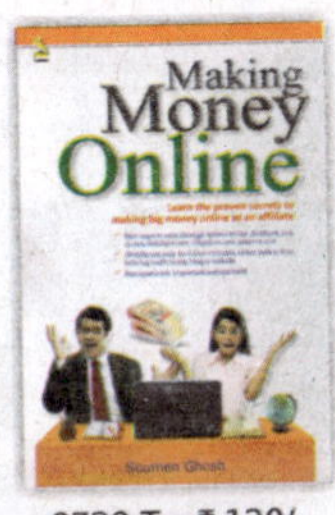

8729 T • ₹ 120/-

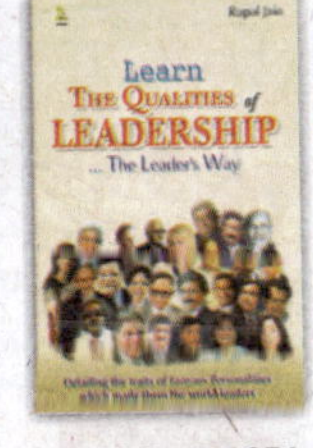

9697 P • ₹ 195/-

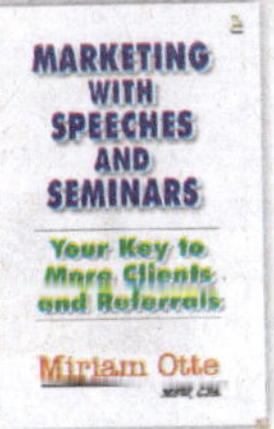

9313 D • ₹ 150/-

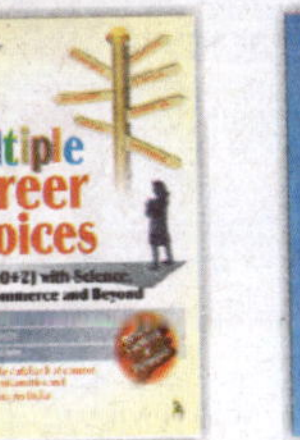

5623 B • ₹ 250/-

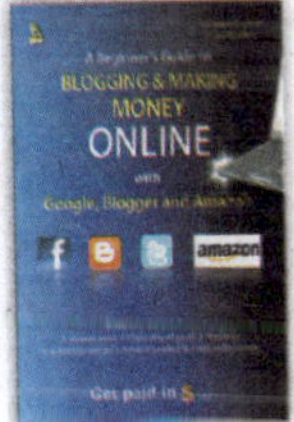

9439 L • ₹ 150/-

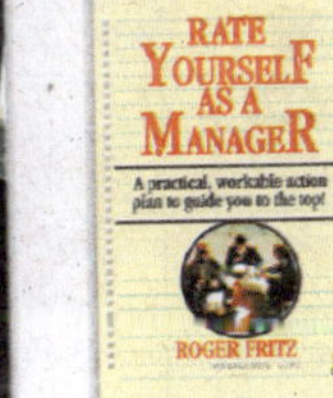

5441 D • ₹ 195/-

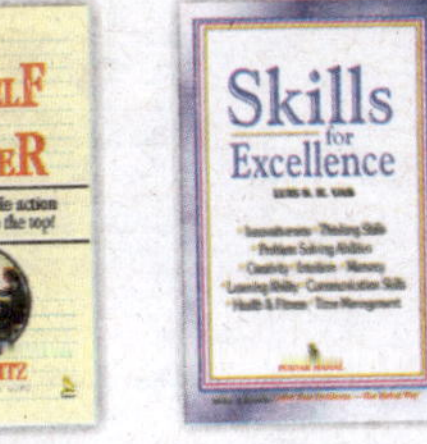

8883 D • ₹ 150/-

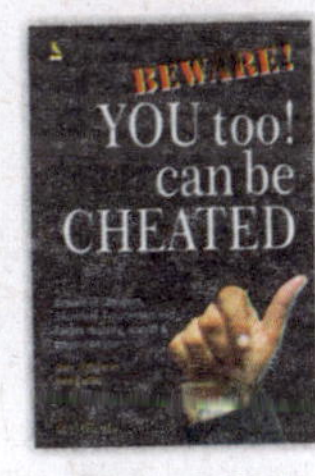

8735 F • ₹ 150/-

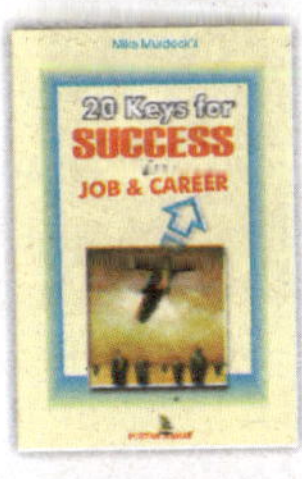

4018 D • ₹ 150/-

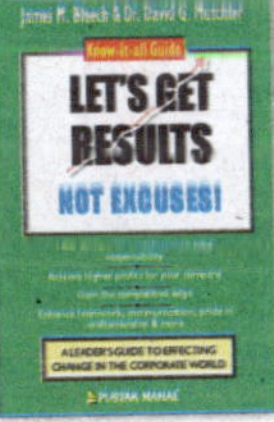

9079 B • ₹ 195/-

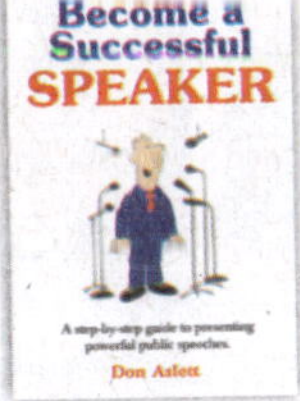

4005 E • ₹ 195/-

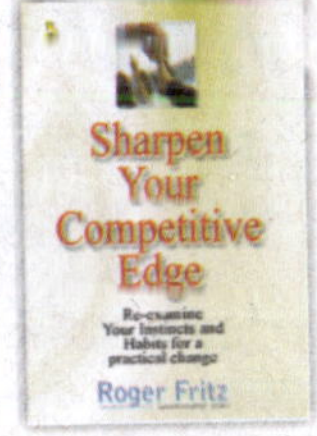

5643 B • ₹ 120/-

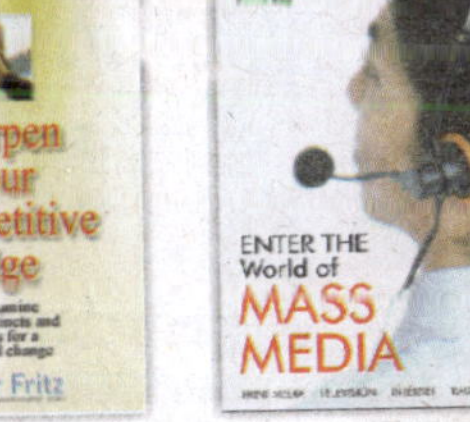

9431 C • ₹ 175/-

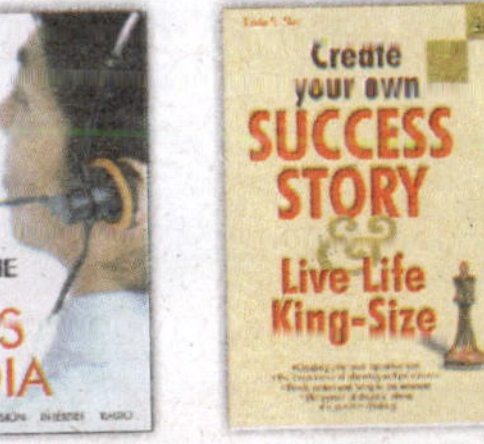

8990 C • ₹ 96/-

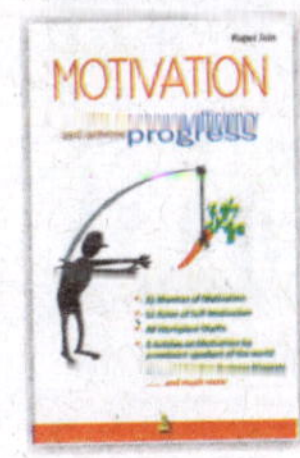

9763 P • Rs. 195/-

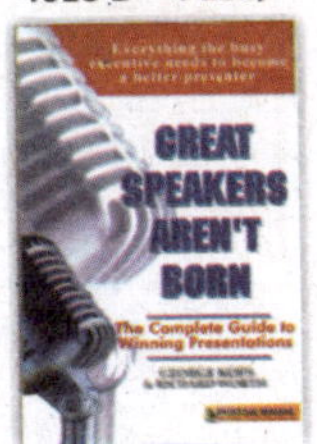

5618 D • ₹ 120/-

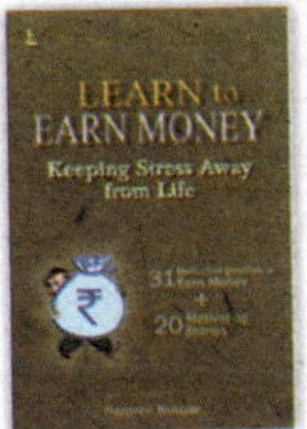

5640 C • ₹ 120/-

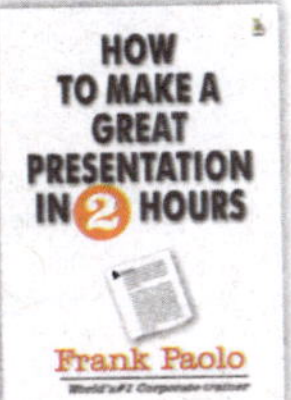

5615 D • ₹ 150/-

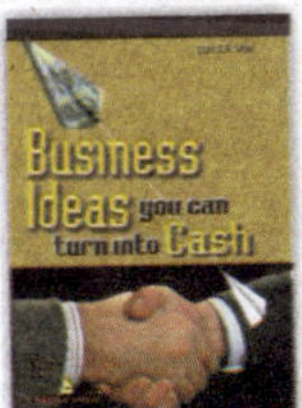

8972 C • ₹ 80/-

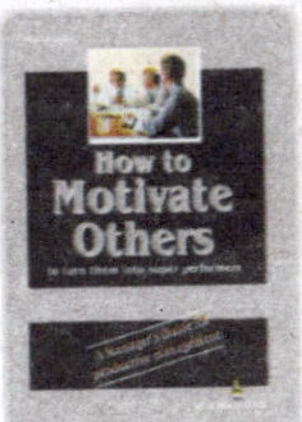

4001 A • ₹ 150/-

5646 A • ₹ 225/-

4017 D • ₹ 150/-

PERSONALITY DEVELOPMENT

8748 E • ₹ 195/-

9666 A • ₹ 150/-

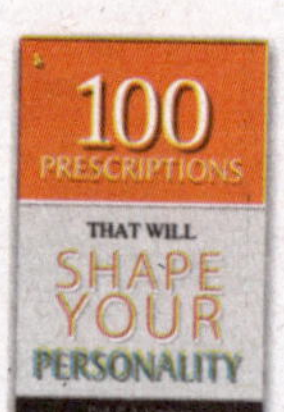
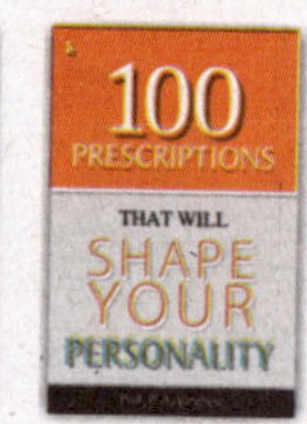

9678 R • ₹ 195/-

9670 E • ₹ 240/-

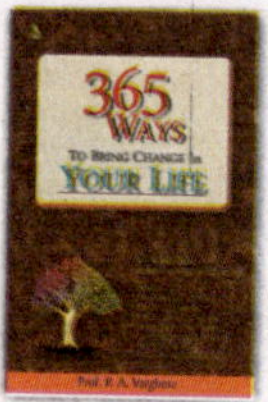

9696 M • ₹ 220/-

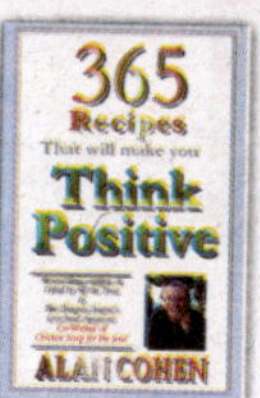

9070 B • ₹ 195/-

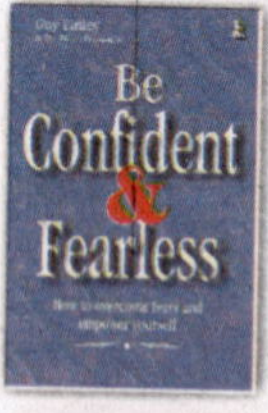

9028 D • ₹ 175/-

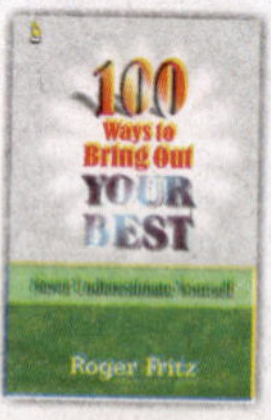

5641 A • ₹ 150/-

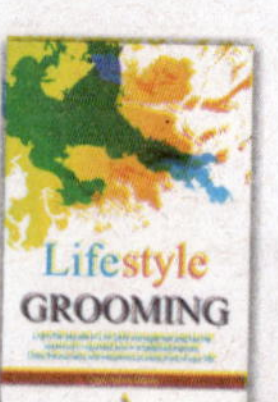

9450 B • ₹ 195/-

9088 C • ₹ 195/-

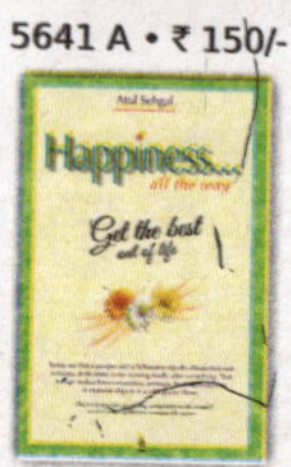

9667 B • ₹ 150/-

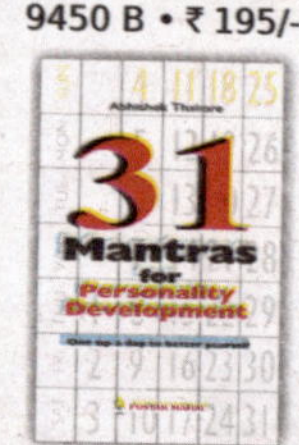

8966 E • ₹ 100/-

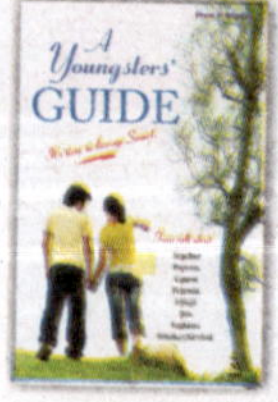

5639 B • ₹ 80/-

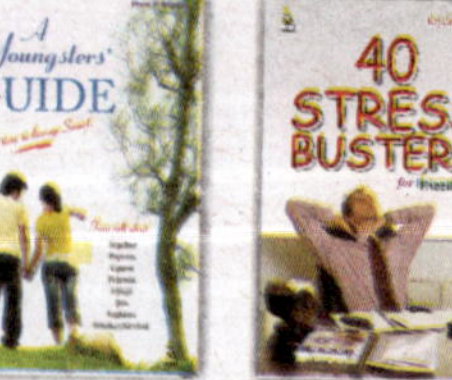
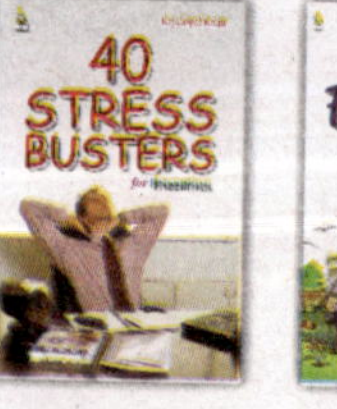

9466 T • ₹ 96/-

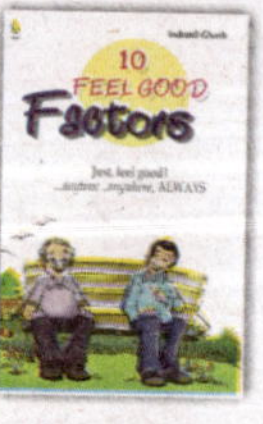

9973 B • ₹ 110/-

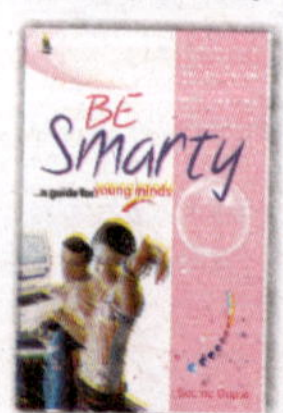

9981 B • ₹ 96/-

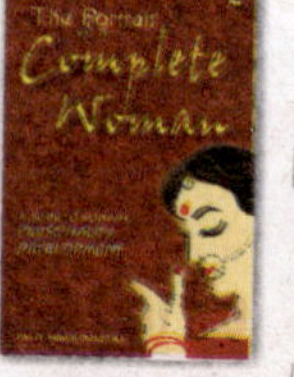

8868 D • ₹ 120/-

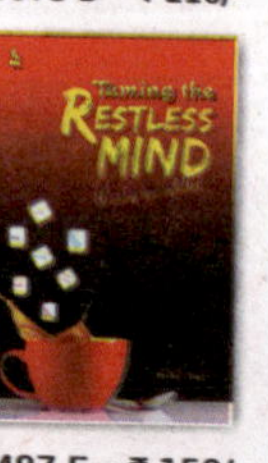

9487 E • ₹ 150/-

STUDENT DEVELOPMENT

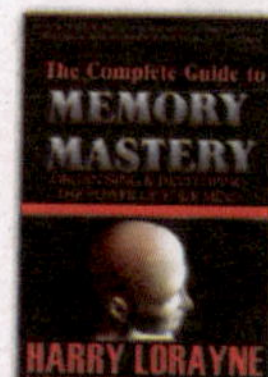

9090 A • ₹ 220/-

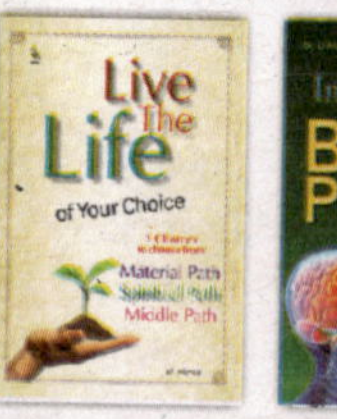

9668 C • ₹ 150/-

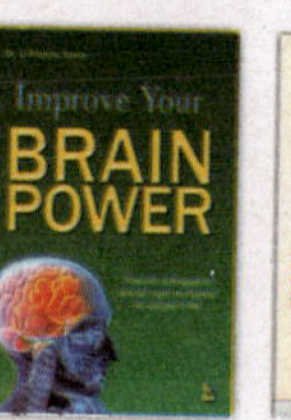

9071 D • ₹ 165/-

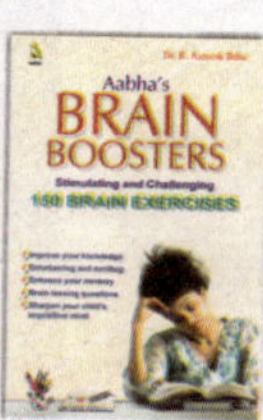

8731 B • ₹ 100/-

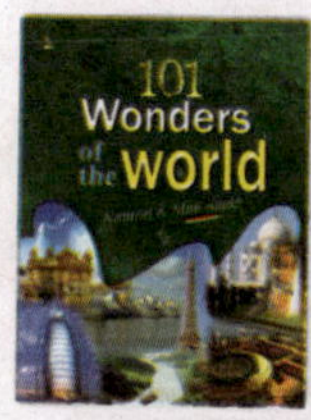

9495 R • ₹ 175/-

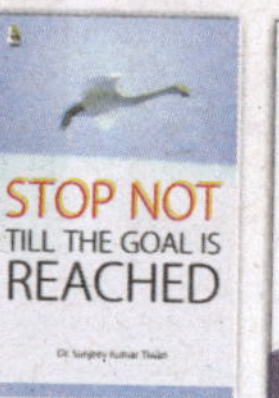

9455 C • ₹ 150/-

5622 A • ₹ 120/-

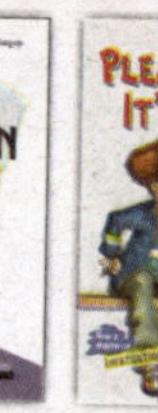

9967 C • ₹ 120/-

2241 J • ₹ 100/-

94441 S • ₹ 195/-

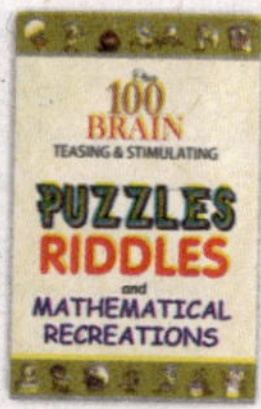
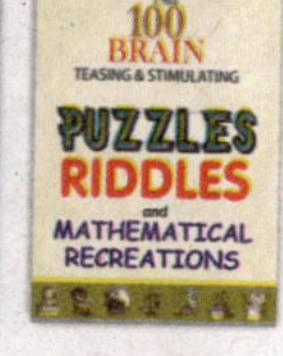

9654 D • ₹ 100/-

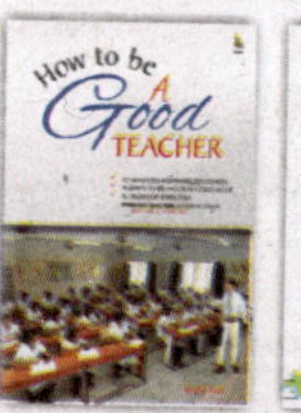

9652 D • ₹ 120/-

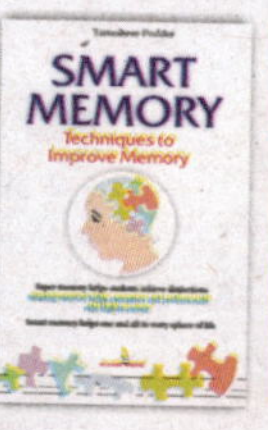

8962 A • ₹ 150/-

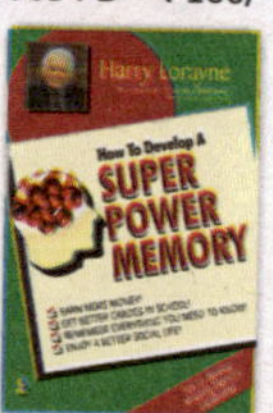

9089 D • ₹ 135/-

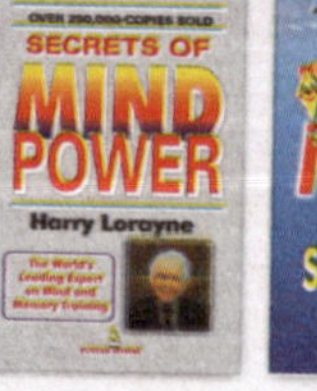

4016 D • ₹ 160/-

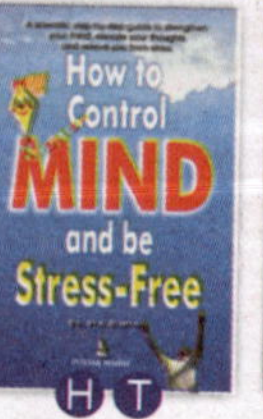

4009 K • ₹ 150/-

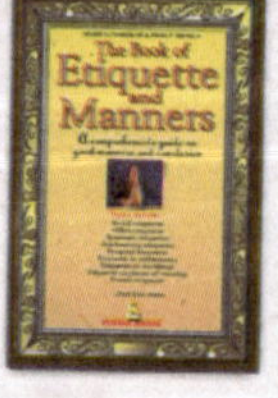

8997 B • ₹ 120/-

4010 L • ₹ 100/-

9787 P • ₹ 100/-

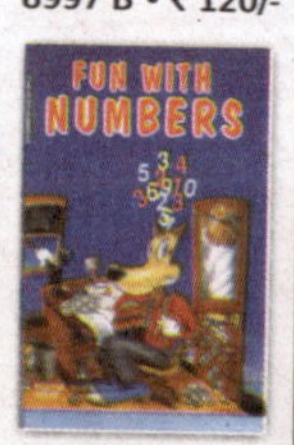

2244 D • ₹ 80/-

PARENTING

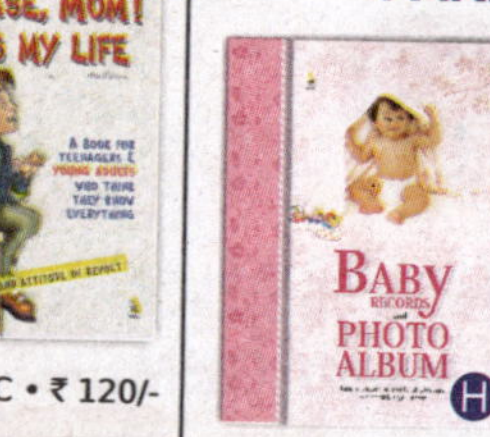

9906 J • ₹ 250/- (HB)

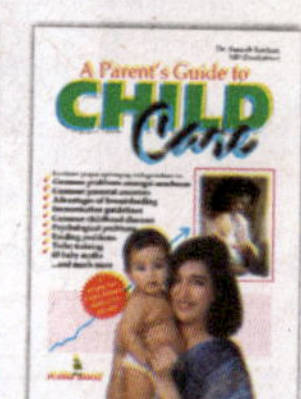

8261 D • ₹ 180/-

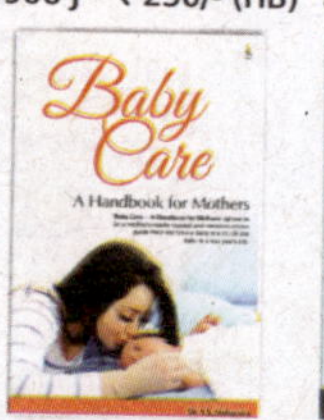

9674 J • ₹ 220/-

9784 J • ₹ 150/-

9594 K • ₹ 80/-

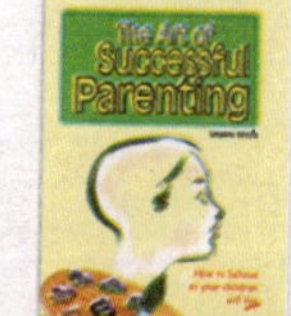

8917 D • ₹ 120/-

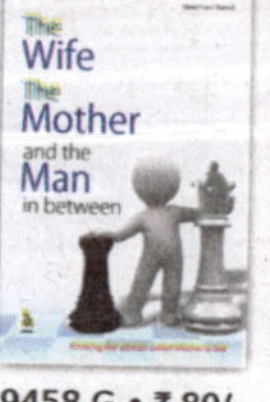

9458 G • ₹ 80/-

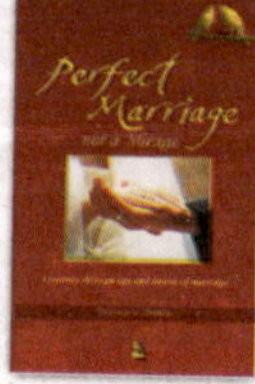

9438 B • ₹ 150/-

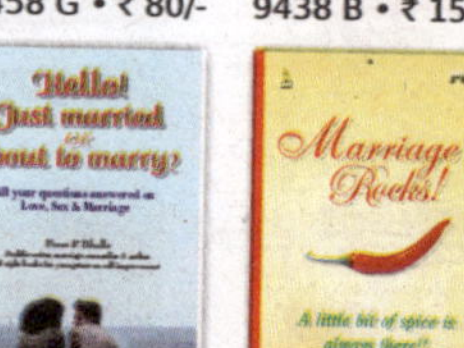

9065 A • ₹ 80/-

9994 E • ₹ 120/-

ALTERNATIVE THERAPIES

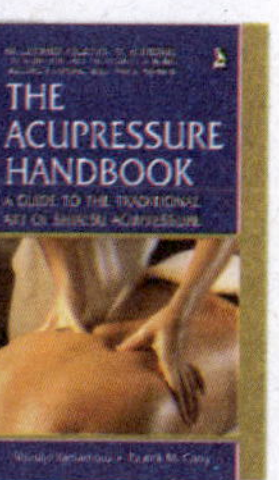

882 F • ₹ 215/-

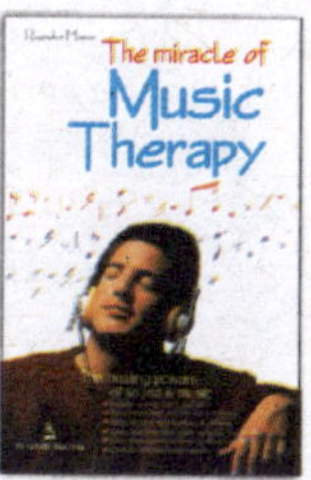

8983 E • ₹ 100/-

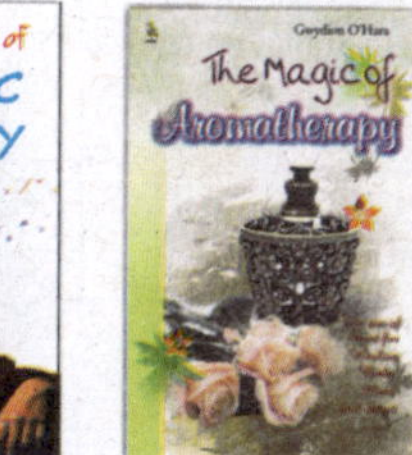

8836 D • ₹ 135/-

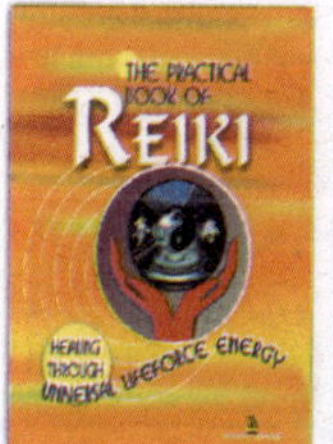

9935 F • ₹ 120/-

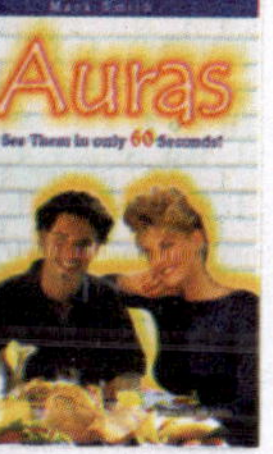

637 D • ₹ 96/-

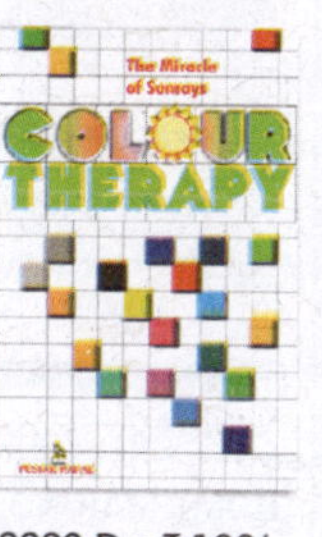

8889 D • ₹ 100/-

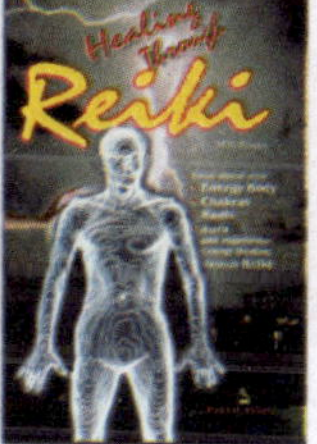

8842 D • ₹ 100/-

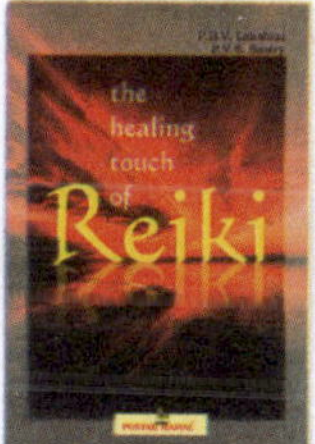

8941 A • ₹ 100/-

COMMON AILMENTS & DISEASES

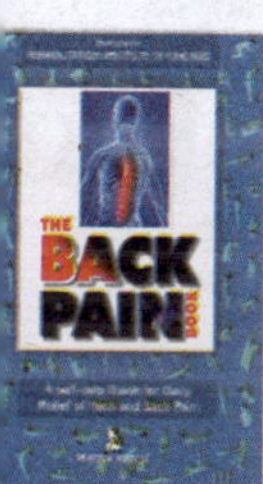

891 D • ₹ 120/-

8281 A • ₹ 100/-

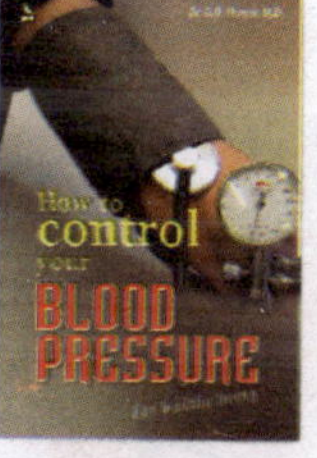

8094 D • ₹ 120/-

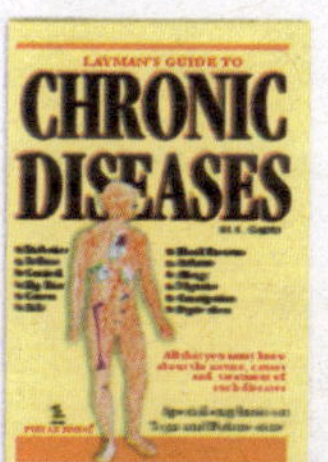

8848 D • ₹ 150/-

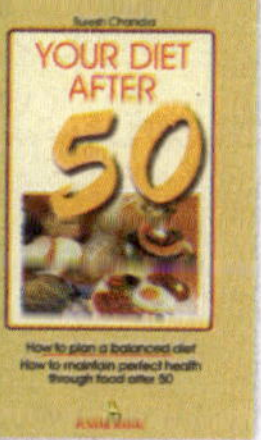

276 A • ₹ 96/-

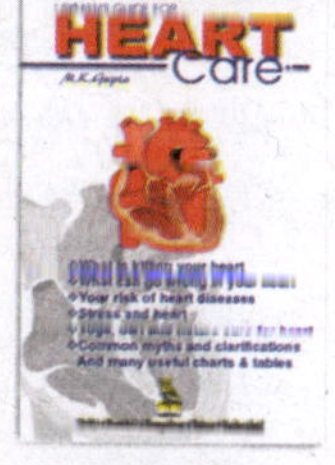

8888 D • ₹ 96/-

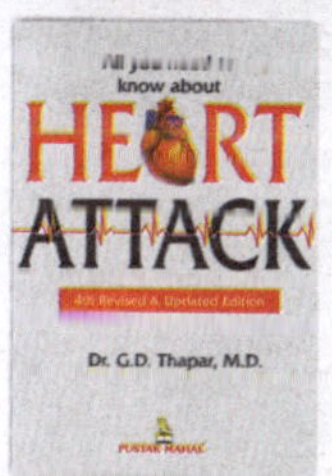

8908 D • ₹ 120/-

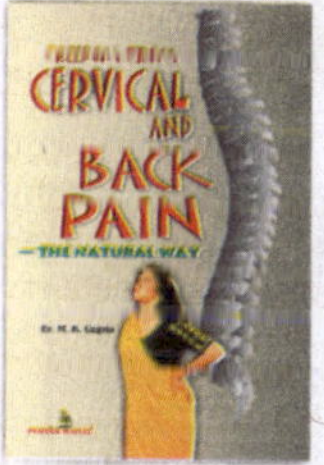

8878 B • ₹ 80/-

GENERAL HEALTH

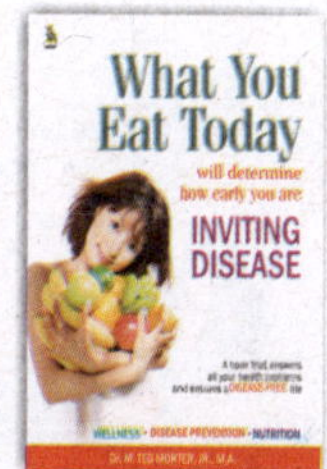

9075 C • ₹ 225/-

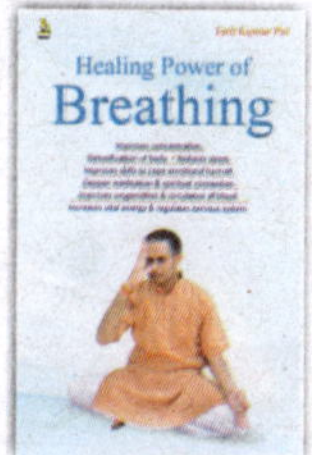

8747 D • ₹ 150/-

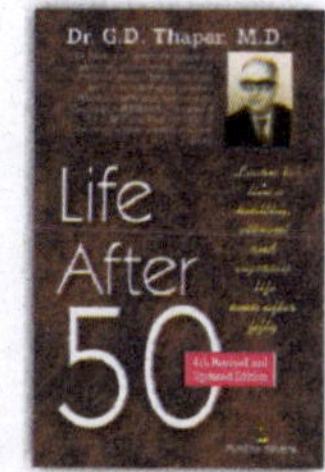

9940 D • ₹ 150/-

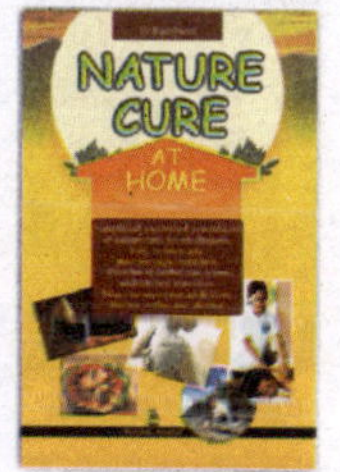

8859 G • ₹ 80/-

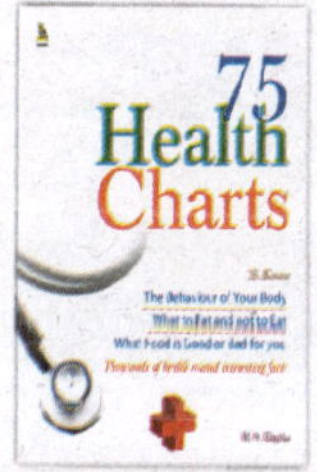

8877 A • ₹ 150/-

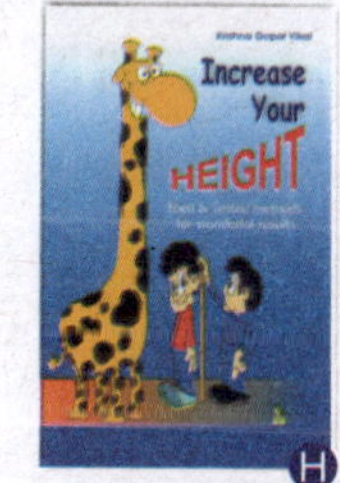

8847 M • ₹ 100/-

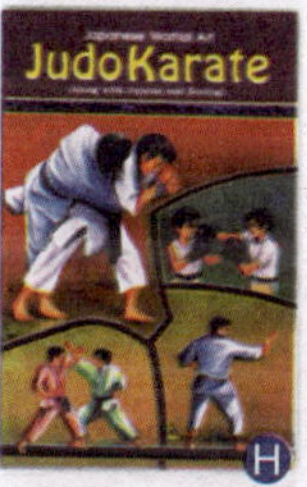

8870 D • ₹ 100/-

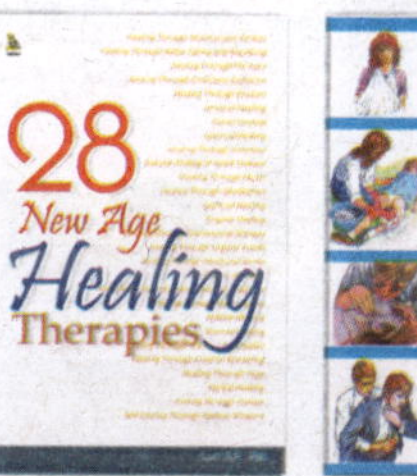

9950 B • ₹ 120/-

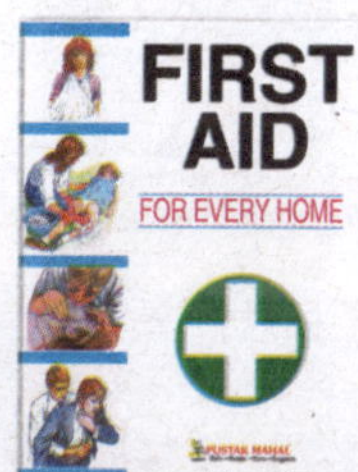

9902 F • ₹ 120/-

SLIMMING & FITNESS

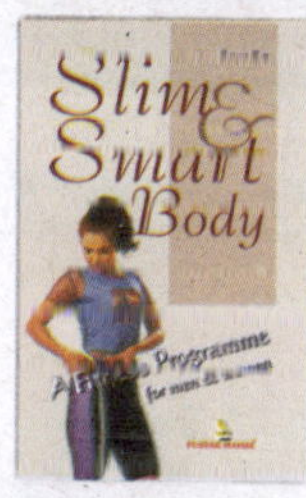

8277 B • ₹ 120/-

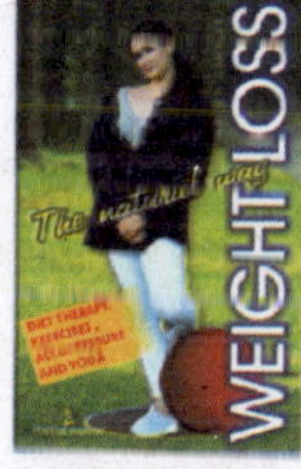

8875 K • ₹ 120/-

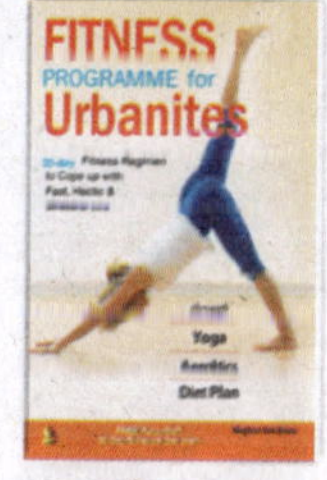

9445 A • ₹ 150/-

DIET & NUTRITION

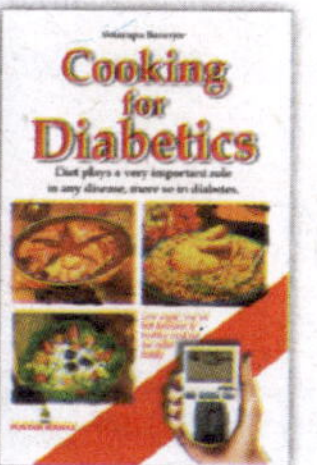

9941 D • ₹ 100/-

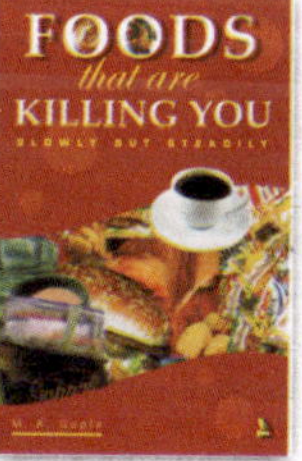

8904 D • ₹ 150/-

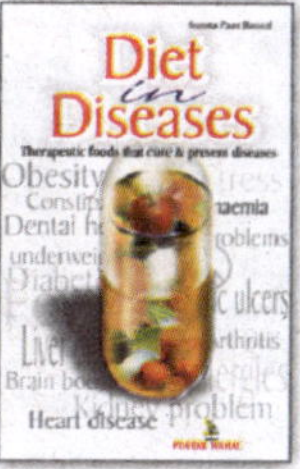

8985 B • ₹ 120/-

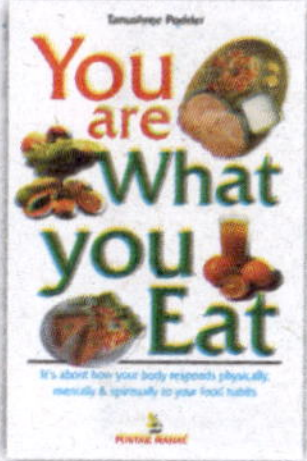

8968 G • ₹ 120/-

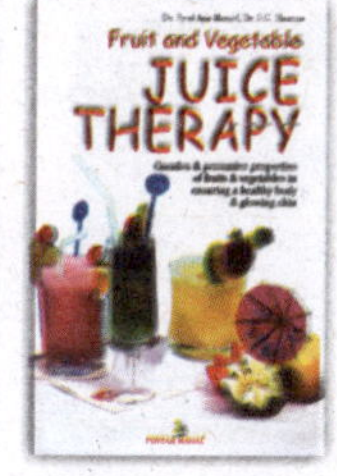

8271 C • ₹ 96/-

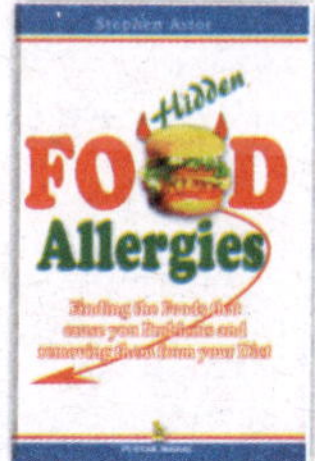

9037 D • ₹ 150/-

HINDOOLOGY / RELIGION / SPIRITUAL BOOKS

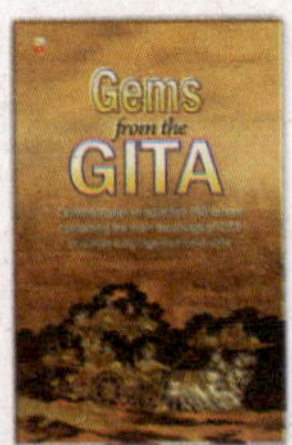

9873 C • ₹ 60/-

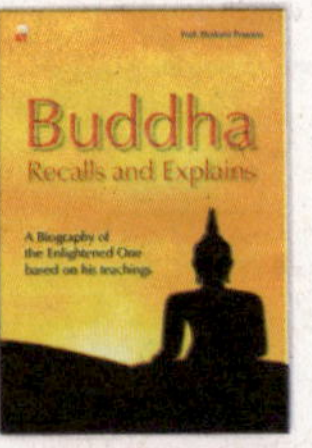

9770 E • ₹ 150/-

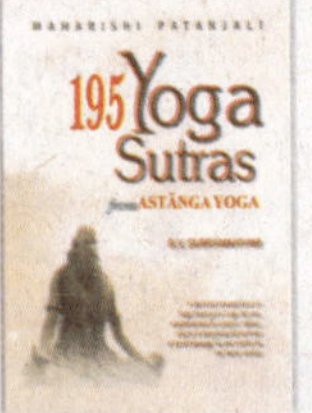

9453 A • ₹ 250/-

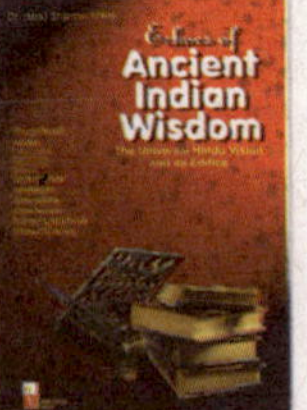

4179 A • ₹ 295/- (HB)

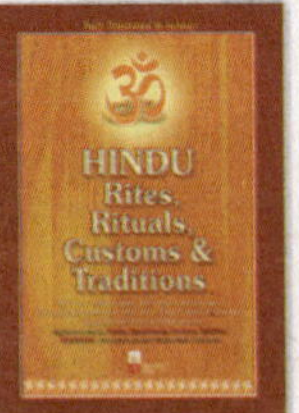

4138 B Rs. 250

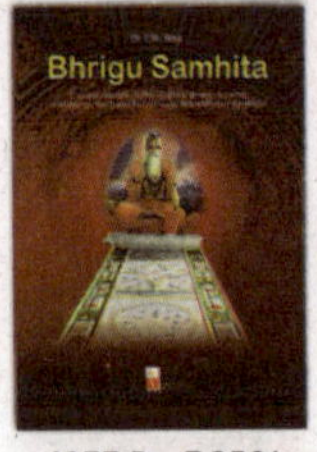

4177 B • ₹ 250/-

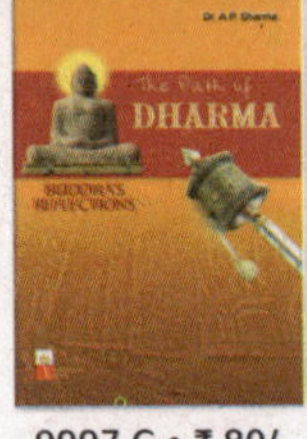

9997 C • ₹ 80/-

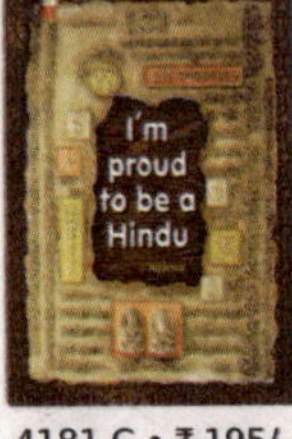

4181 C • ₹ 195/-

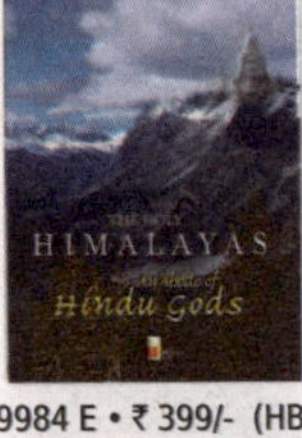

9984 E • ₹ 399/- (HB)

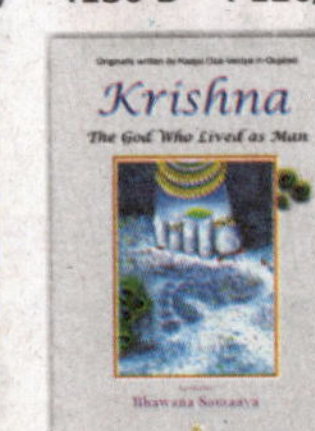
4130 B • ₹ 120/-

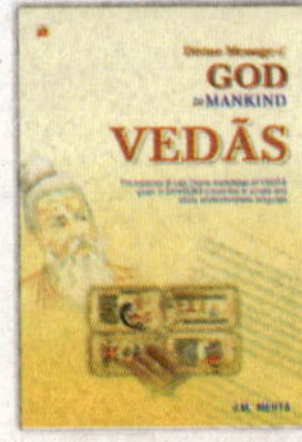

9811 P • ₹ 120/-

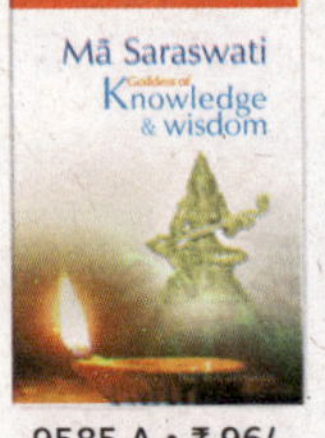

9585 A • ₹ 96/-

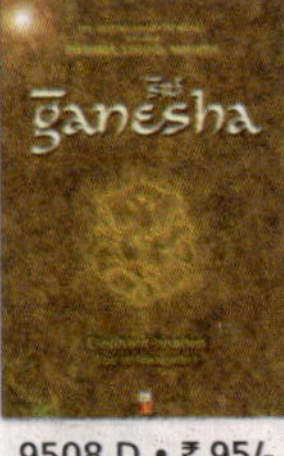

9508 D • ₹ 95/-

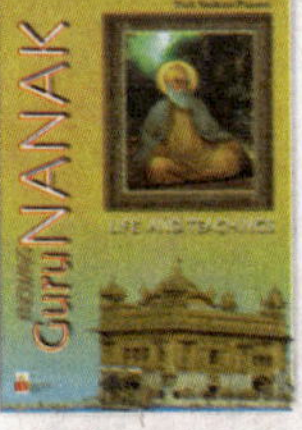

9989 D • ₹ 96/-

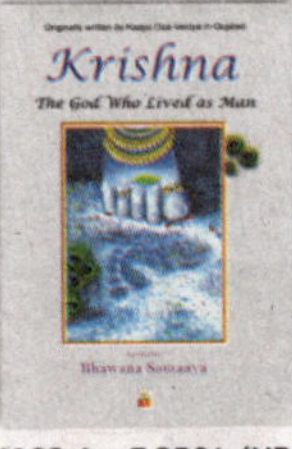

4183 A • ₹ 350/- (HB)

9504 D • ₹ 100/-

9540 D • ₹ 150/-

9513 A • ₹ 195/-

4126 B • ₹ 96/-

9812 R • ₹ 120/-

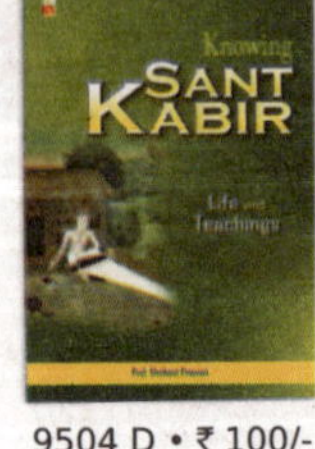

9504 D • ₹ 100/-

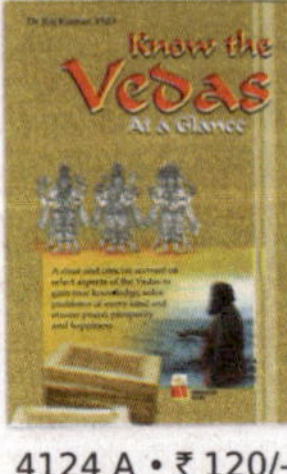

4124 A • ₹ 120/-

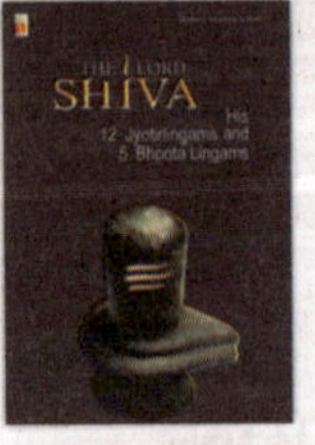

4190 C • ₹ 160/-

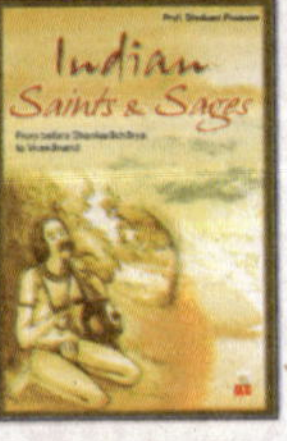

9509 A • ₹ 150/-

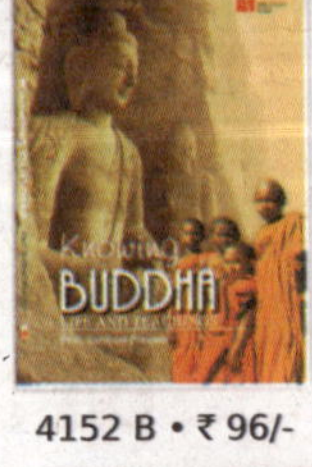

4152 B • ₹ 96/-

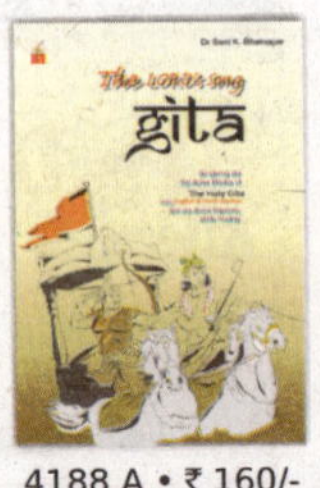

4188 A • ₹ 160/-

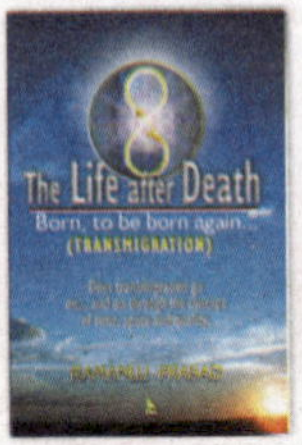

4132 D • ₹ 100/-

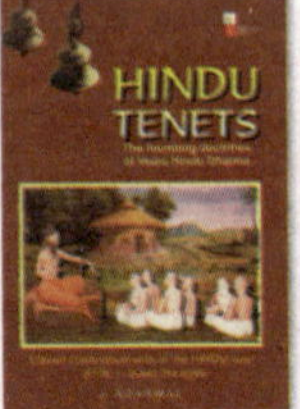

9987 E • ₹ 150/-

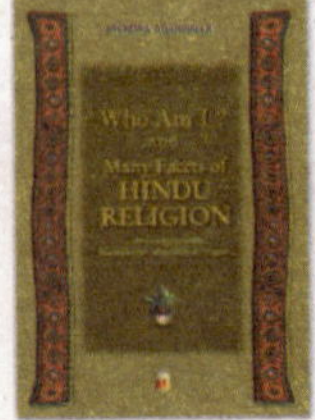
9520 D • ₹ 120/-

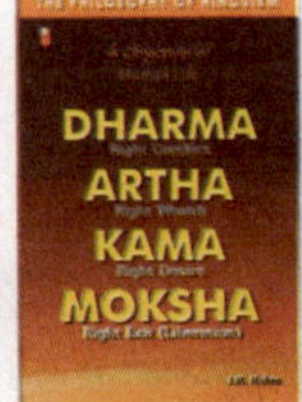

4134 B • ₹ 80/-

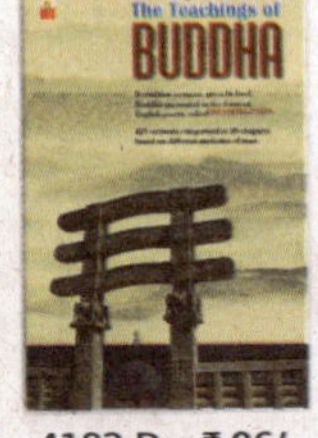

4182 D • ₹ 96/-

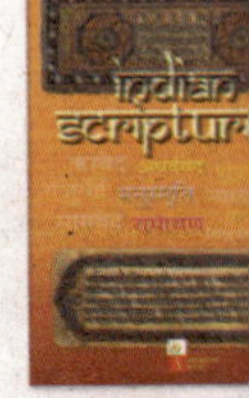
9405 A • ₹ 1

COMPUTERS

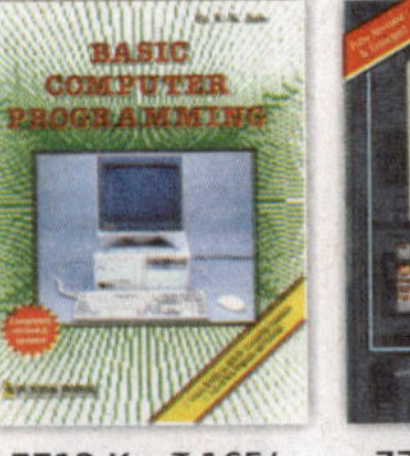

7712 K • ₹ 165/-

7711 J • ₹ 12

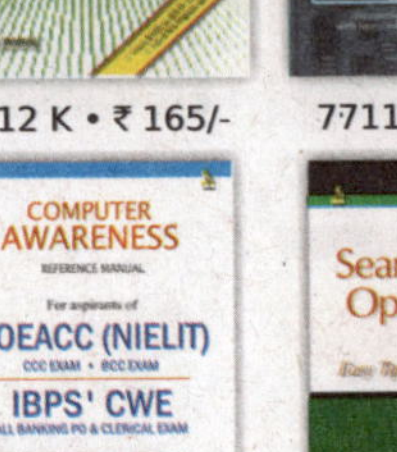

9768 C • ₹ 175/-

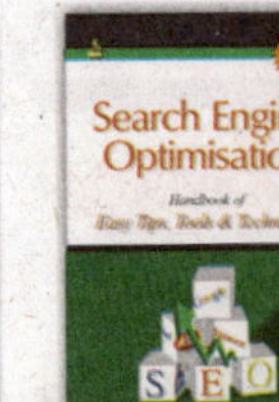

7766 A • ₹ 12

HOME MAKING / GRILLS & RAILI

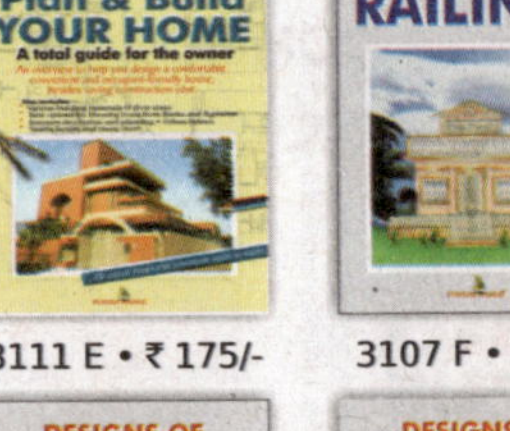

3111 E • ₹ 175/-

3107 F • ₹ 8

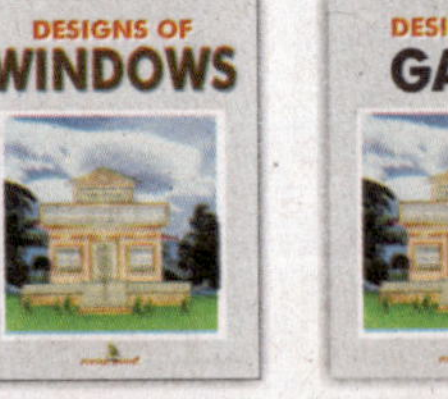

3106 E • ₹ 100/-

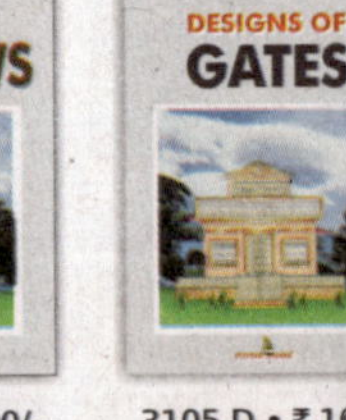

3105 D • ₹ 1

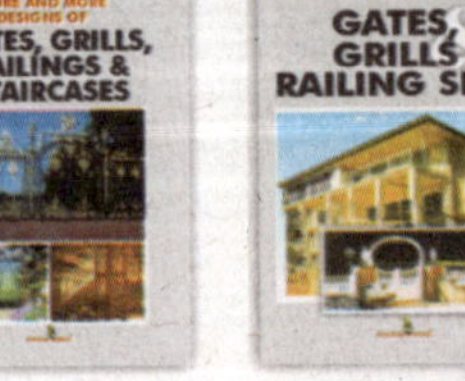

3108 G • ₹ 150/-

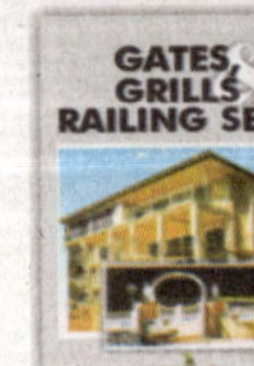
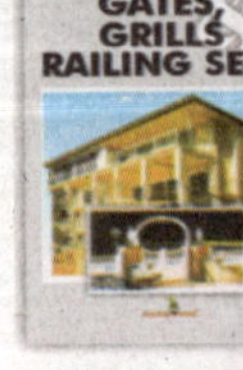
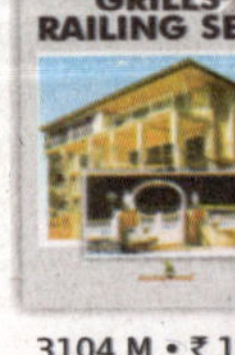

3104 M • ₹ 1

ASTROLOGY/VASTU/HYPNOTISM/PAMISTRY

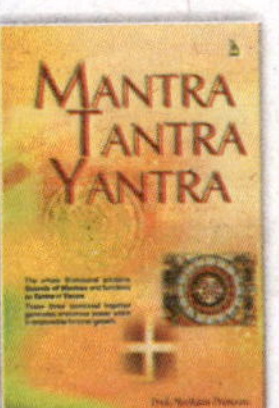
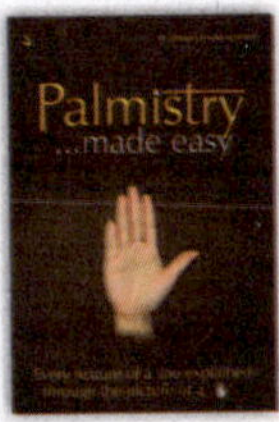
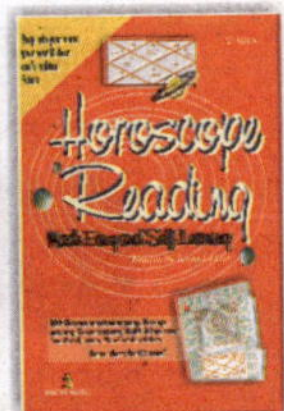
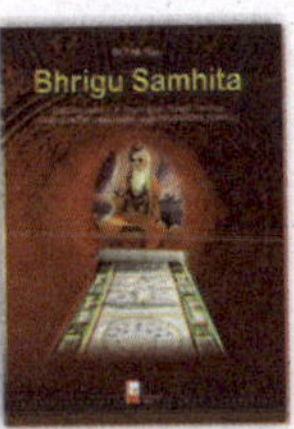
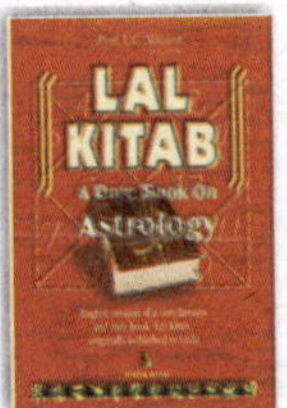

9871 A • ₹ 240/- 9693 H • ₹ 195/- 9671 F • ₹ 195/- 2127 D • ₹ 250/- 4177 C • ₹ 295/- 9086 A • ₹ 295/-HB

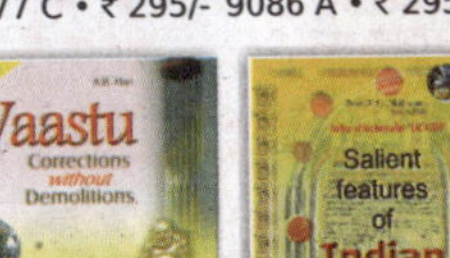
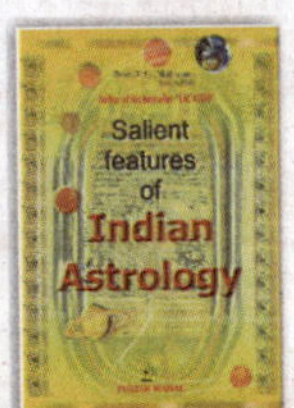
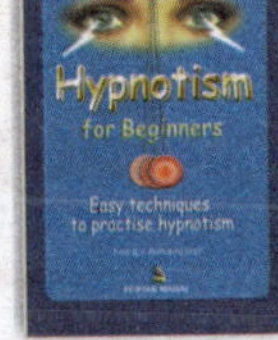
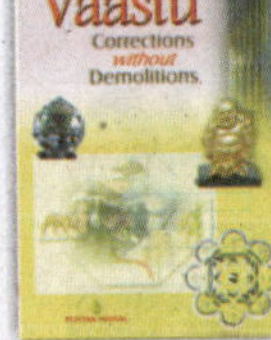

2116 D • ₹ 150/- 8259 D • ₹ 88/ 2109 F • ₹ 150/- 2112 D • ₹ 120/- 3110 B • ₹ 120/- 2133 B • ₹ 96/-

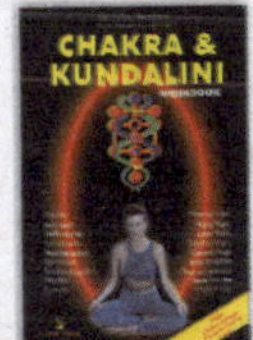
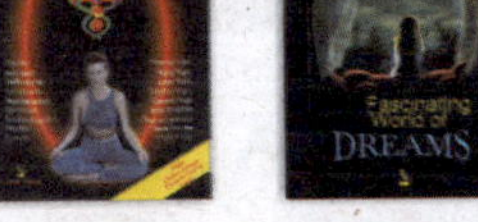
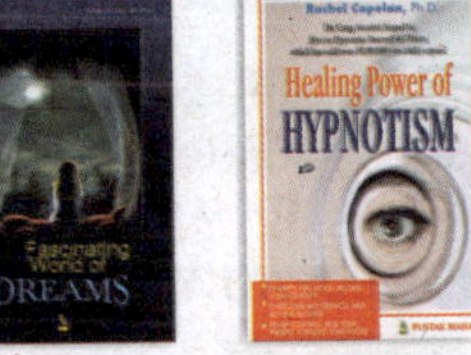
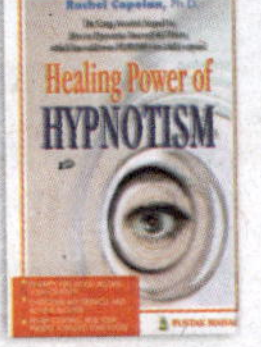
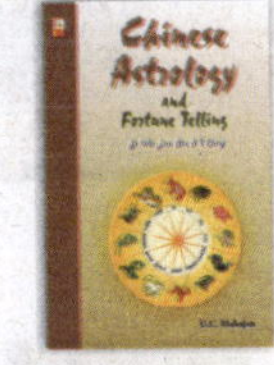
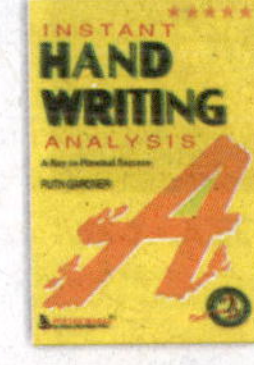
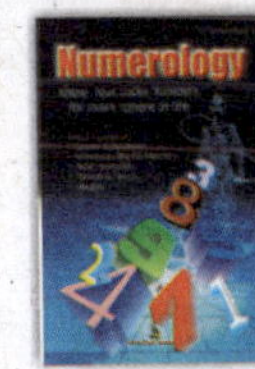

8899 D • ₹ 195/- 8925 D • ₹ 96/- 2132 A • ₹ 150/- 9432 D • ₹ 150/- 2120 D • ₹ 150/- 2109 F • ₹ 100/-

ENGLISH IMPROVEMENT

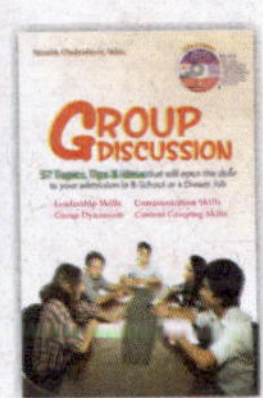
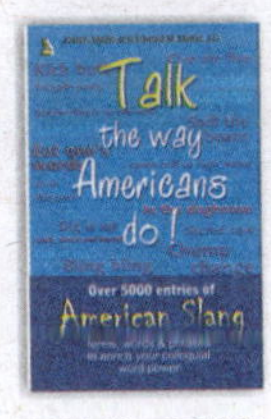
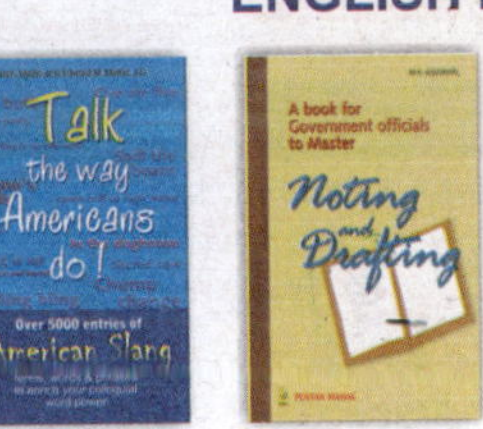
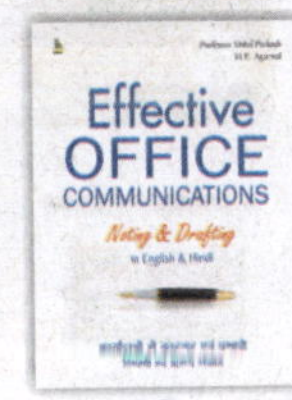
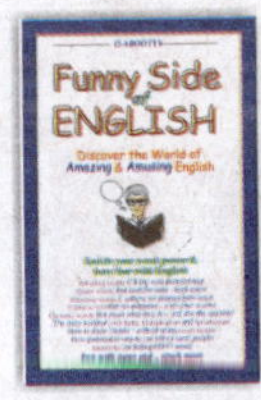
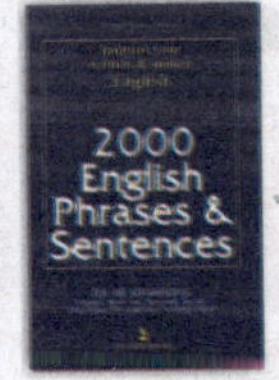

97540 D • ₹ 175/- 5541 C • ₹ 190/ 6651 E • ₹ 195/- 9448 D • ₹ 175/- 9056 A • ₹ 125/- 5538 D • ₹ 100/-

PERSON & PERSONALITIES

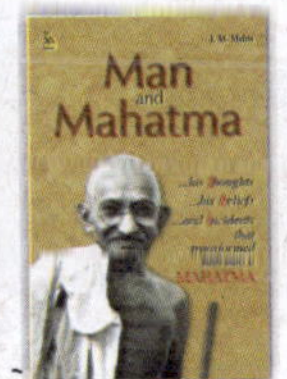
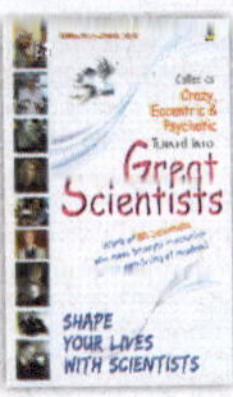
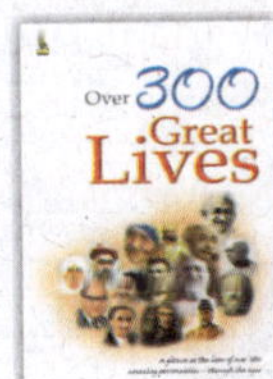
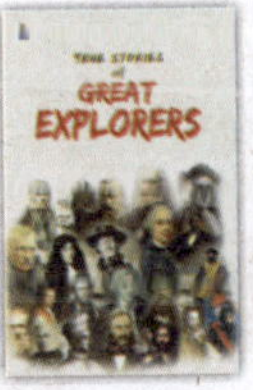
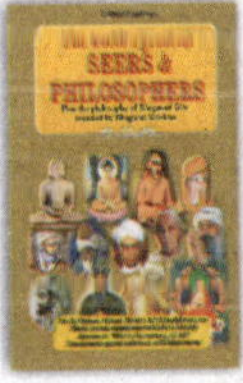
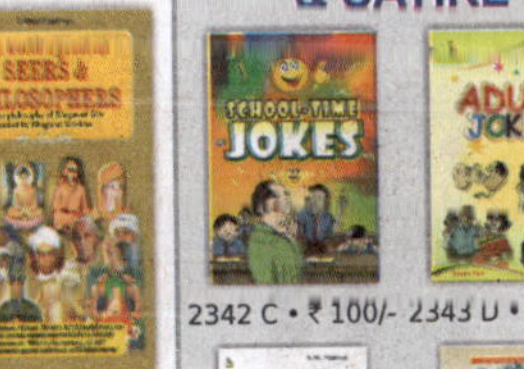
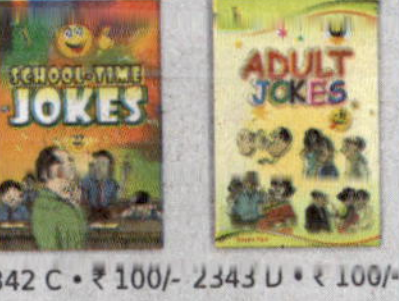

9669 D • ₹ 120/- 9825 E • ₹ 150/- 2113 D • ₹ 195/- 9764 R • ₹ 100/- 8991 D • ₹ 120/-

BODY/BEAUTY CARE

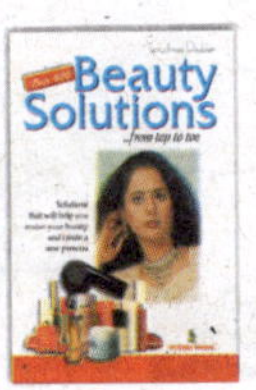
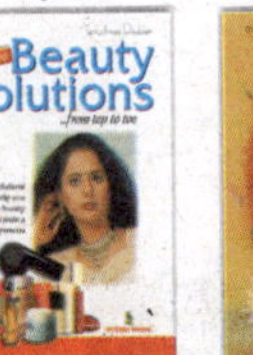
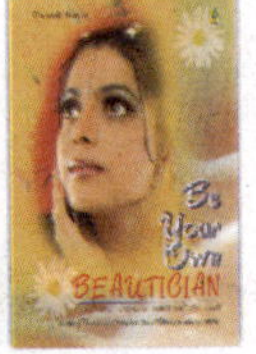
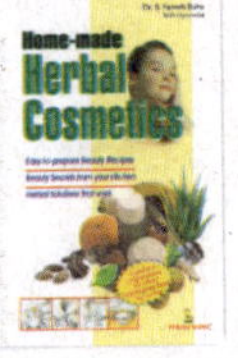
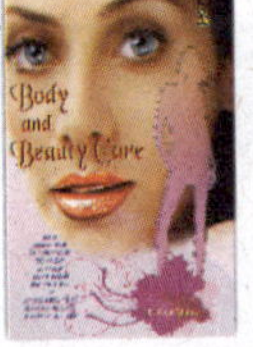
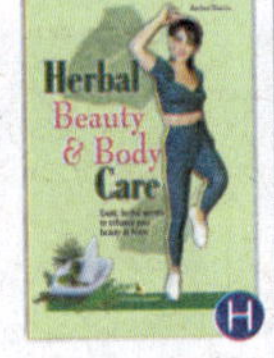
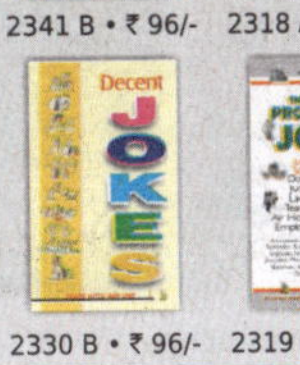

8093 D • ₹ 150/- 9986 B • ₹ 150/- 8971 B • ₹ 120/- 9922 F • ₹ 120/- 8865 F • ₹ 120/-

JOKES HUMOUR & SATIRE

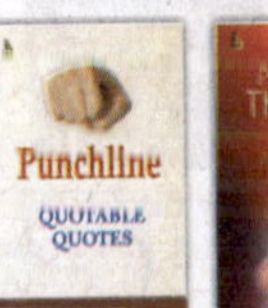
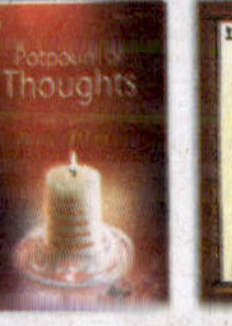

2342 C • ₹ 100/- 2343 D • ₹ 100/-

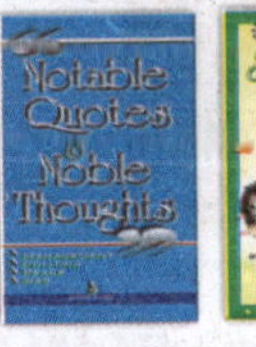
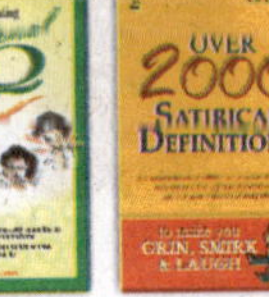

2341 B • ₹ 96/- 2318 A • ₹ 96/-

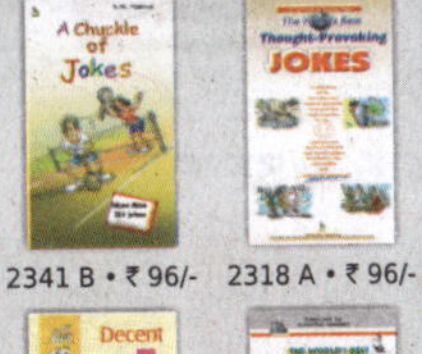
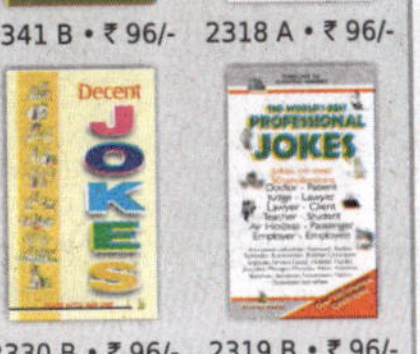

2330 B • ₹ 96/- 2319 B • ₹ 96/-

FICTION

FIVE BOOKS

Set Price ₹ 495/- ₹ 99/- Each Volume

Set Code SH 001

THREE BOOKS

Set Price ₹ 297/- ₹ 99/- Each Volume

Set Code 9795 A

THREE BOOKS

Set Code 9752 B • ₹ 550/-

SAYING/QUOTATIONS/PROVERBS

9474 F • ₹ 170/- 9789 A • ₹ 150/- 8999 D • ₹ 80/-

9953 A • ₹ 100/- 8947 E • ₹ 100/- 8890 D • ₹ 150/-

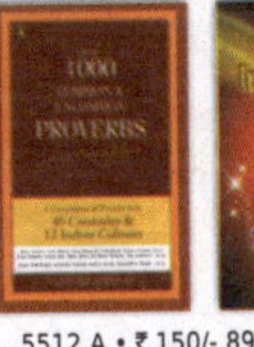
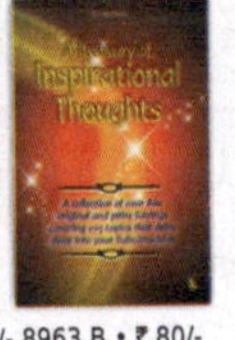
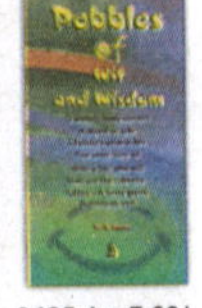

5512 A • ₹ 150/- 8963 B • ₹ 80/- 9425 A • ₹ 60/-

FUN, FACTS, MAGIC & MYSTERIES

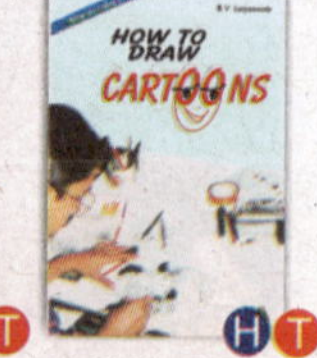
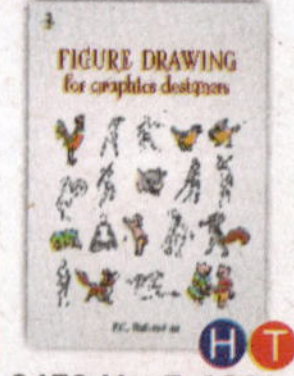
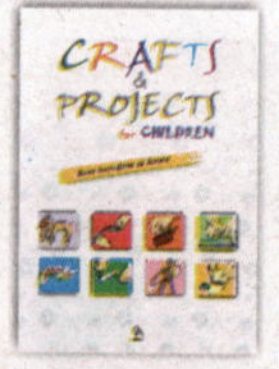
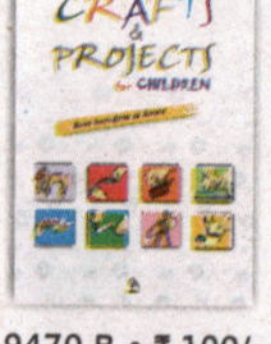
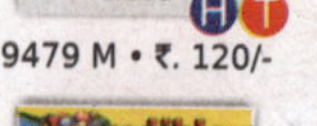

9484 B • ₹ 150/- | 2275 D • ₹ 120/- | 9479 M • ₹. 120/- | 9470 B • ₹ 100/-

2208 M • ₹ 100/- | 9816 D • ₹ 100/- | 2247 F • ₹ 100/- | 2250 A • ₹ 110/-

2211 F • ₹ 100/- | 9457 E • ₹ 150/- | 2237 M • ₹ 100/- | 2335 A • ₹ 80/-

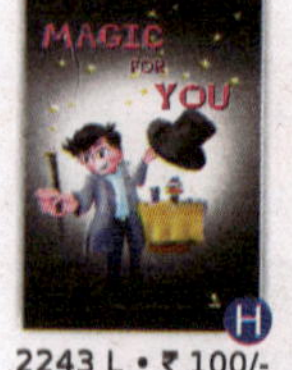
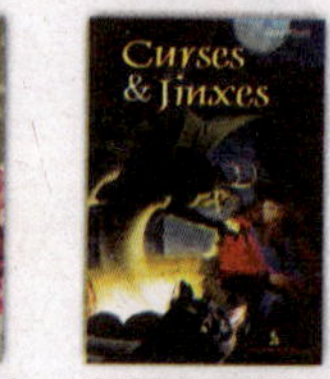
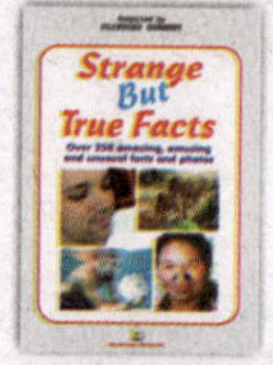
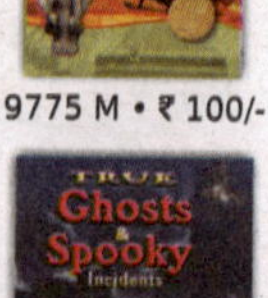

2243 L • ₹ 100/- | 9775 M • ₹ 100/- | 9985 A • ₹ 80/- | 5110 A • ₹ 80/-

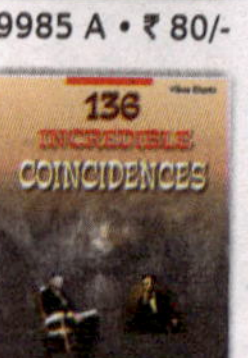
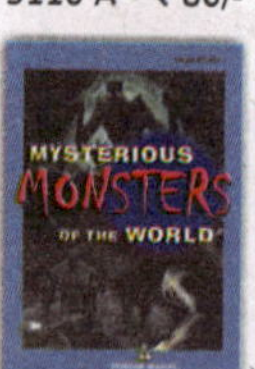
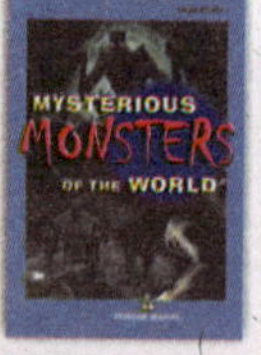

2337 C • ₹ 100/- | 2336 B • ₹ 100/- | 2331 C • ₹ 100/- | 9977 B • ₹ 100/-

YOGA & MEDITATION

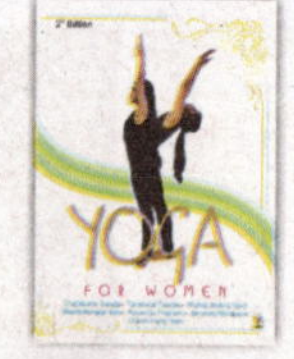
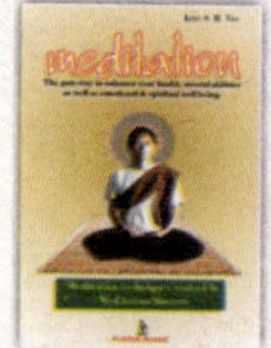

8269 A • ₹ 195/- | 9998 D • ₹ 150/- | 8939 D • ₹ 96/-

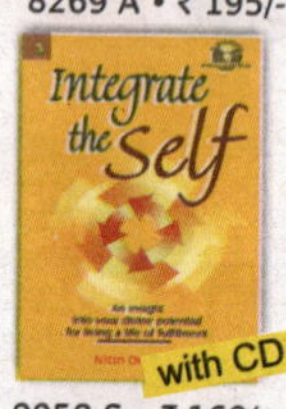

9958 S • ₹ 160/- | 9087 B • ₹ 195/- | 2118 F • ₹ 120/-

8901 D • ₹ 150/- | 8099 D • ₹ 80/- | 9025 D • ₹ 80/-

HOMEOPATHY, AYURDEDA

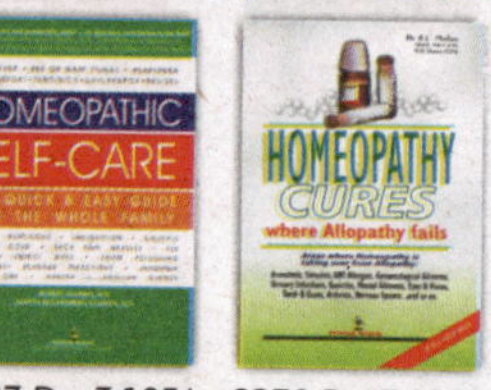

9446 B • ₹ 150/- | 8887 D • ₹ 195/- | 8270 B • ₹ 195/- | 8923 D • ₹ 195/-

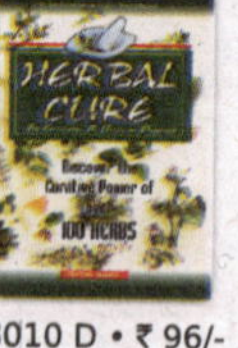
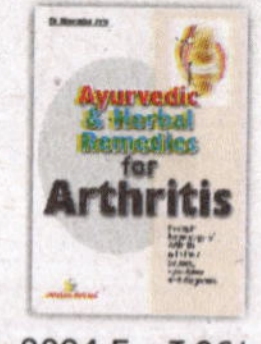
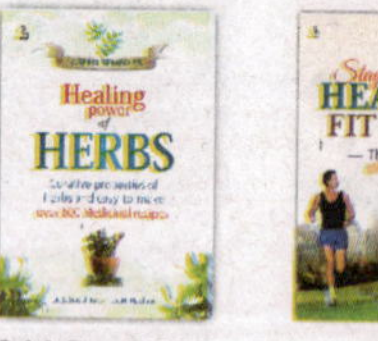
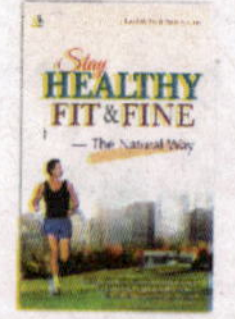

8010 D • ₹ 96/- | 9094 E • ₹ 96/- | 8944 D • ₹ 175/- | 8948 A • ₹ 120/-

WORLD FAMOUS SERIES

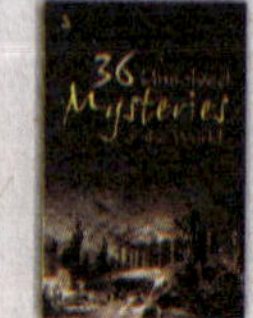
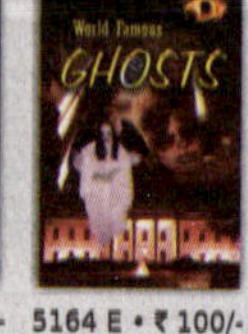
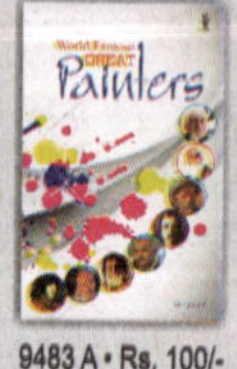
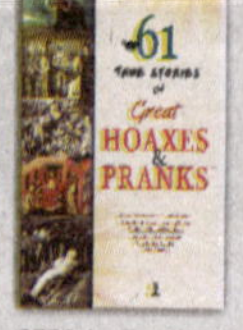
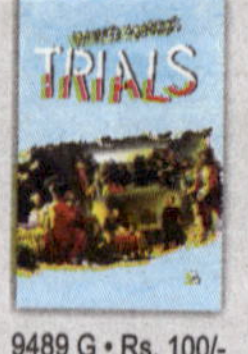
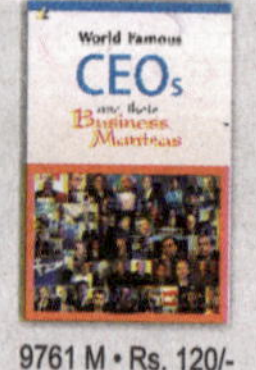

9472 D • ₹ 100/- | 5164 E • ₹ 100/- | 9483 A • Rs. 100/- | 51107 • ₹ 100/- | 9766 A • Rs. 100/- | 9489 G • Rs. 100/- | 9761 M • Rs. 120/-

World Famous Mysterious Objects
True Stories of Mowglis and other Wild Childrens
World Famous Treasures (Lost and Found)
World Famous WARs & Battles
True Stories of Mystic Places
World Famous Adventures
World Famous Military Operations
World Famous Spy Scandals
World Famous Spies & Spymasters
World Famous Crooks & Con Men
True Stories 81 Weird Humans
True Stories of Great Explorers
World Famous Strange Mysteries
and many more.......

LOVE, ROMANCE & SEX

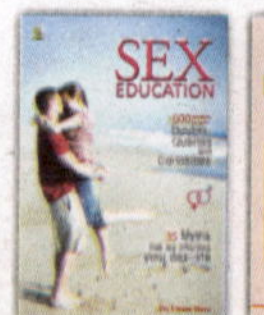
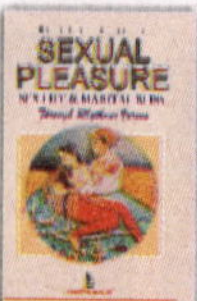
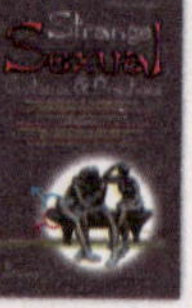
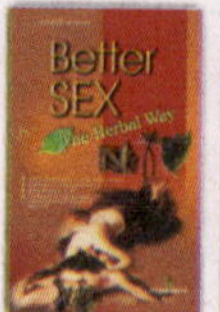
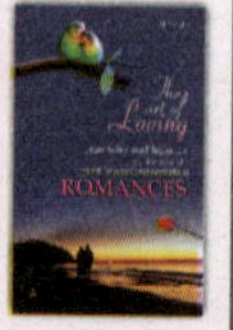

9602 B • Rs. 125/- | 8260 D • Rs. 96/- | 8266 D • Rs. 80/- | 8278 C • Rs. 100/- | 8916 D • Rs. 120/-

MORAL, WISDOM & FAIRY TALES

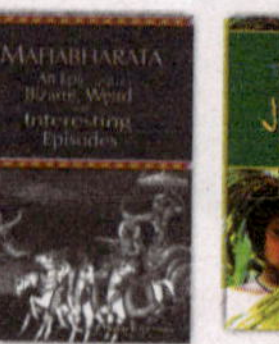
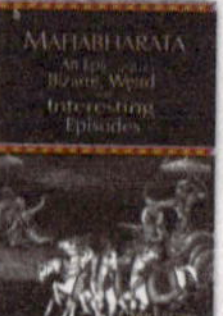
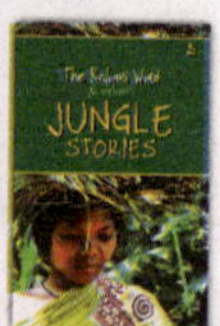
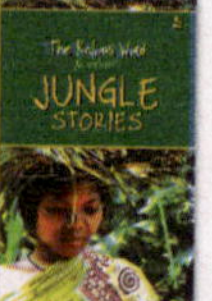
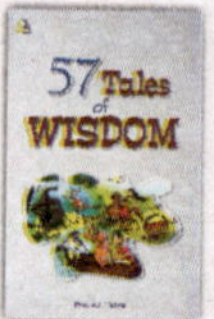
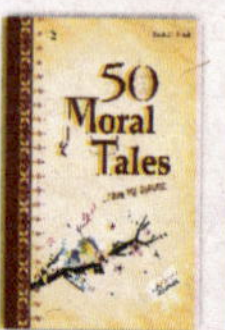
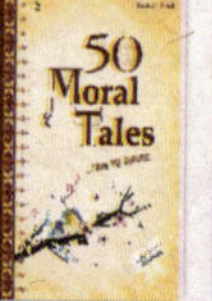
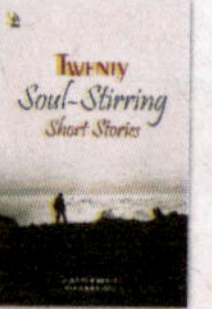
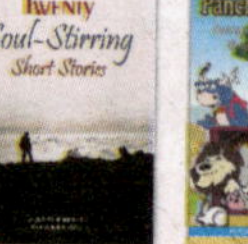
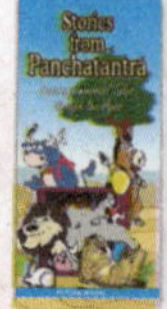

9677 P • Rs. 150/- | 9486 D • Rs. 250/- | 8967 F • Rs. 80/- | 9077 E • Rs.120/- | 9563 N • Rs. 125/- | 2289 D • ₹ 96/-